GW00542504

The Alkaline Solution

—

Surviving the Modern Western Diet

HOW ACID-BASE BALANCE AND MAGNESIUM
DEFICIENCY IMPACTS DIABETES, HEART DISEASE,
DEPRESSION, MIGRAINES, CANCER
AND PAIN MANAGEMENT

Professor Jürgen Vormann & Peter Ochsenham

Professor Jürgen Vormann & Peter Ochsenham
/madhouseMEDIA

Published by www.madhousemedia.com.au

The Alkaline Solution - Survive the Modern Western Diet. How acid-base balance and magnesium deficiency impact: diabetes, heart disease, depression, migraine, cancer and pain management —1st ed.

Contents

[1] Foreword 1

[2] And You Thought it was Simple 3

[3] How the Body Establishes a Balance 8

[4] On the Trail of the Causes of Osteoporosis.......... 16

[5] The Chemistry Behind Osteoporosis................... 19

[6] Understanding Alkalinity 23

[7] The Role of Protein... 26

[8] A Study Tells the Story.. 30

[9] A Different Understanding of Chronic Pain 34

[10] Acidosis and Alzheimer's 43

[11] The Cancer Connection 46

[12] Acid-base Balance and Metabolic Diseases........ 49

[13] Assessing the Effect of Diet............................... 56

[14] Are Your Adrenals at Risk? How an Alkaline Diet May Help
.... 60

[15] Why Supplementation with Alkaline Minerals Makes Sense
.... 64

[16] Magnesium – Life's Essential Mineral............... 68

[17] The Main Physiological Functions of Magnesium 69

[18] How Magnesium Works 71

[19] How Magnesium is Absorbed by the Body 74

[20] How to Recognise Magnesium Deficiency......................... 82

[21] Your Heart and Brain are at Risk 86

[22] Magnesium and Diabetes.. 90

[23] Magnesium and Neurological Issues 97

[24] Magnesium and Pregnancy... 103

[25] Other Benefits of Magnesium for Women 106

[26] When Magnesium is the Wrong Thing to Give............. 107

[27] Do You Have a Magnesium Deficiency? 109

[28] How to Select the Best Magnesium Supplement............. 111

[29] Conclusion 116

Appendix 1 Magnesium Deficiency Metabolic Typing.......... 118

Appendix 2: Youtube Video Resources: Magnesium Deficiency

Questions Answered By Professor Vormann: 129

Bibliography 131

Acknowledgments 142

About The Authors.. 143

All truth passes through three stages.
First, it is ridiculed.
Second, it is violently opposed.
Third, it is accepted as being self-evident.

—Arthur Schopenhauer

[1]

Foreword

The modern western diet is a testament to our affluence but has also become a major contributor to ill health and chronic disease. As recently as twenty years ago, the medical establishment, at the coal face of service delivery, doubted there was any close correlation between diet and disease. However, researchers were uncovering a very different picture.

We fear the same is happening today. We now postulate that in Australia magnesium is under prescribed by medical doctors, even though the research is very strong and undeniable for numerous conditions. Unfortunately, there seems to be a blind spot to the use of magnesium.

If we look at an over acid diet, for example, our fear is that the understanding and recognition of its impact on health will go unnoticed by the people that can make a change in the population.

We hope this book serves as a reminder that the data is out there, that change can happen, and that it gives you what you need to make modifications in your diet that may even save your life.

[2]

And You Thought it was Simple

There has been much of information disseminated on what is known as the "Paleo diet", which our ancestors are said to have consumed during that period of human history when we were hunter-gatherers.

Paleo is short for the Paleolithic Era, the period of roughly two and a half million years that preceded the agricultural revolution. The term "Paleolithic" is made up of two Greek words. *Paleo* comes from *palaios*, meaning old—referring to prehistoric times—and *lithos* from the Greek word for stone. Hence, we commonly refer to the period when our ancestors were hunter-gatherers as the Stone Age, since it was marked by the development and use of such items as stone-tipped arrows for hunting.

For about the last 8,500 to 10,000 years, depending on which part of the globe we are talking about, humans have been cultivating crops and breeding livestock. When we say "livestock", we use the term in the more general sense that includes not only cattle but also foods, such as poultry and farmed seafood. Before the development of agriculture, all of our food was a product of the wild (Cordain et al., 2005).

Many of us have known for a long time that most of our modern diseases are intimately linked to the industrial world's flawed eating habits. From cardiovascular issues, such as heart disease, stroke, and congestive heart failure, to diabetes, cancer, osteoporosis, and autoimmune diseases, such as Crohn's or rheumatoid arthritis. If whole populations began to eat wild berries, roots, nuts, free-range meats and wild seafood, much of the pharmaceutical industry and the medical field—the areas that deal with degenerative diseases— would quite simply go out of business.

Despite the current popularity of a return to what people imagine as the diet our Stone Age ancestors feasted on, it isn't quite so simple as cutting out grains and other starchy carbohydrates, along with replacing the mass-produced factory-farmed meat most of us consume with grass-fed beef and poultry, wild-caught fish, pasture-raised eggs, and other products. For whether we are talking about Australia or China, the United States or the countries that make up the European Union, Canada or Japan, our foods today just aren't the same as those of the Paleolithic era.

It isn't simply a matter of "a cow is a cow is a cow." A modern cow has been bred to be a very different creature from those killed and consumed by our hunter-gatherer ancestors. Consequently, what we consume—even when we try for the most natural of diets today—has a quite different effect on our metabolism, and we should keep in mind that this kind of Paleolithic diet cannot feed the more than eight billion people on earth.

Don't get us wrong. We're all for cleaning up our diet. We are saying that simply opting for more naturally produced foods isn't enough. Neither is it merely a matter of adding vitamins and minerals to our diet, whether as additives, such as vitamin D added to milk or taking supplements. Many do all these things yet still don't get well, let alone enjoy optimum health. Millions are tired, overweight, anxious, and in many cases suffer from anything from haemorrhoids to acne. Food alone isn't the answer for most of us living in the modern world.

What has been lacking is the scientific data showing why this is so. Now, at last, this data is available. From this scientific research, we are now finally able to say definitively what the issues are and figure out how to fix them. When you see the data, you'll understand why it isn't quite so straightforward as merely changing our diet.

This is what's different about this book—it gives you the hard science, which no one has ever done in a book of this kind before.

To understand the fundamental difference between a Paleolithic diet and what most of us eat today, it's necessary to consider the findings of an elaborate scientific study that investigated 159 possible preagricultural diets.

You didn't know there were that many Paleo diets? Most think there is essentially just one diet. We said it was more complicated than just switching from grains and factory farmed beef!

One of the most crucial aspects of the human metabolism has to do with the balance of acid versus alkaline throughout our system—with the exception of our digestive system. In science, we generally refer to this as the "acid-base" balance, the term "base" denoting alkaline.

The study we referred to earlier set out to discover the effect of these 159 possible Paleo diets on the acid-base balance of the human body (Sebastian et al., 2002). The researchers sought to determine the net endogenous acid production from such diets.

The word "endogenous" is important. We aren't so much concerned with the alkaline or acidic nature of a food in itself, but with what the body does with a particular food. For instance, lemons are an example of an acidic food that, in the body, has an alkaline effect. That's because the digestive system takes what we put into our mouths and breaks it down into its components. It's the overall result of digestion that impacts our health.

Extreme acidity can be dangerous. You wouldn't put your finger into concentrated hydrochloric acid (HCl)—or at least, you would only ever do it once! But during our evolution, our taste has developed in such a way that we like some acidity in our food, such as the use of vinegar or lemon juice. Other healthy ingredients are often combined with "acid tasting" foodstuffs. As we don't have taste receptors for alkalinity, we can taste only the free acid in a food. So, overall our tongue doesn't help us in deciding what kind of food is acid or alkaline, in terms of our metabolism.

Regarding the acid produced in the human body, the majority of the 159 preagricultural diets resulted in an excess of alkaline over acid. Relatively few of the diets resulted in an excess of acid. Why is this significant?

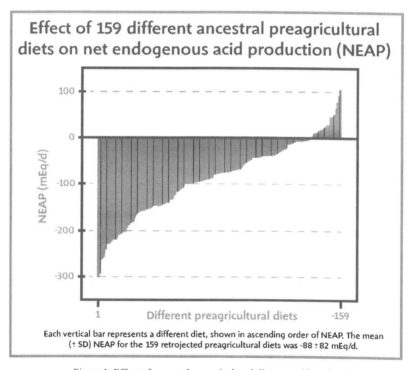

Figure 1: Effect of ancestral preagricultural diets on acid production

If we examine a typical modern Western diet, we find that the result in terms of the acid-alkaline balance (acid-base, to be more correct) is fundamentally different from that of the foods ingested by Stone Age humans. To get a little technical for just a moment, so that you understand what we are up against when we talk about switching to a Paleo diet. If you calculate the mean net endogenous production, the preagricultural diets exhibited -88+/-[VJ1]82 mEq/d (milliequivalents per day). That's quite a surplus on the alkaline side. What it means for us today is that, if we take into consideration our long preagricultural ancestry, we are genetically equipped to consume an alkaline surplus in our diet.

What do we get from our food? In contrast to our Stone Age ancestors, we currently get an acid surplus—and quite a large surplus at that. This is a fundamental shift, and it has great bearing when it comes to understanding the causes of many of our modern diseases.

Allow us to tell you about the research conducted by the Swedish nutritionist Ragnar Berg, who worked in the city of Dresden, Germany, as the Director of the Johannesstadt Hospital for Nutritional Physiology. The most significant aspect of his extensive testing involved the absorption and excretion of minerals in his patients. He was one of the first—this was as far back as the beginning of the 20th century—to say "consistently healthy human nutrition must contain a greater amount of bases than acids."

Dr. Berg's investigation of this topic led to the use of alkaline minerals as a complementary therapy for a broad variety of diseases. Ever since then, at least in Germany, the basic therapies in natural medicine have emphasised the importance of the acid-base balance. In fact, the first products created for this purpose entered the market as far back as 1930. It's a well-established complementary therapy in Germany—and yet little known in Australia, the Americas, and in fact much of the modern world.

[3]

How the Body Establishes a Balance

The acid-base balance of the body is referred to as "pH balance." The body doesn't allow the pH balance of our bodies to vary beyond a hair's breadth. Indeed, we have intricate mechanisms to regulate the alkalinity of our bodies.

The main acid-base regulatory mechanism is the blood's ability to buffer against an excess of acid. Over the short-term, we can also excrete acid through the lungs. However, simply breathing doesn't provide a net excretion. To achieve a net excretion, we need the kidneys, which filter the blood and are therefore the most important organs when it comes to regulating the acid-base balance.

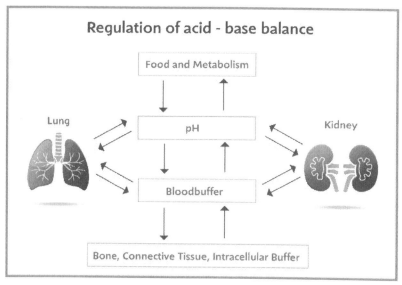

Figure 2: Regulation of acid – base balance

Given that the body can produce its own acids, why do we need to excrete acid? The simple answer is that when we ingest too many acidic foods and beverages, the body can't tolerate the surplus. It therefore works hard to excrete the excess. However, when there is a sustained high input of acid, because of consuming too many acidic substances, the regulatory system is simply unable to fully compensate. This leads to a state commonly referred to as "acidosis". Too much physical activity, especially in athletes who train to extremes, is also a problem. Such excessive activity fosters a state of acidosis, with concurrent negative effects.

What is it about our diet that results in an excess of acid? The Western diet provides an acid load that comes primarily from proteins. But the solution isn't simply, "let's eat less protein so that we can achieve an acid-base homeostasis." We need protein, especially the right kind—as we'll explain.

The main problem is that we eat far too many neutral foods, which are unable to compensate for an acid load, accompanied by insufficient alkaline foods. By alkaline, we are referring to vegetables, most fruits, and salad. The average Western diet is simply woefully lacking in an adequate supply of these foodstuffs.

To understand the chemistry of proteins a little better, the main acidity comes from the sulfur-containing amino acids, which are methionine and cysteine. As these amino acids are metabolised, we must somehow eliminate the sulfur they contain, since the body is incapable of reusing it. The only biochemical means we have of excreting sulfur is to produce sulfuric acid. This is the main dietary source of our acid load, along with the phosphoric acid from soft drinks (soda and fizzy drinks).

We are living in an era when much of Western civilisation enjoys a superabundance of foodstuffs, which for no small number of us leads to wanting to lose weight, especially fat. It's important to understand that all forms of low-calorie dieting—and in the extreme, fasting—metabolise fatty acids into keto acids (commonly known as "ketones"), which have a significant negative impact on our overall acid-base balance. As an aside, most people don't realise that during the time they are losing weight, they are also reducing their acid buffering capacity.

The body is equipped to excrete acid, but the problem is that our kidneys function less and less efficiently as we age. Beginning somewhere between the ages of twenty and thirty, every year we lose about one percent of our kidney function. This results in a significant impact on our acid-base balance, so that we slide slowly into a more acidic state (Frassetto and Sebastian, 1996).

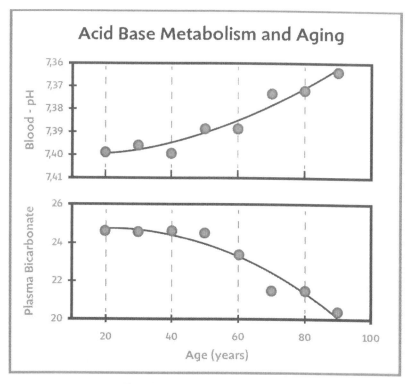

Figure 3: Acid base metabolism and ageing

This occurrence can only be determined from larger populations studies, not by examining a single individual. If we test the pH of a single individual, we will likely conclude that the person is more or less in the right zone. Studying a lone individual is unlikely to reveal changes that are as minute as 0.01 pH units.

Not only does pH change slightly, but also the main blood buffer. Although our bicarbonate levels, which do the buffering, remain relatively stable until around age fifty, following which we see a significant drop.

Some years ago, we did a study of elderly women and men in Sweden who completed a 24-hour urine test to investigate the net acid excretion when the participants ingested a typical Western diet. The mean turned out to be a 60-milliequivalent surplus of acid (Rylander et al., 2006)

Again, thinking back to our preagricultural ancestors, our body chemistry is adapted for an alkaline surplus in the region of 80 milliequivalents. This means we are ingesting a huge amount more acid than we were accustomed to over the course of a few million years.

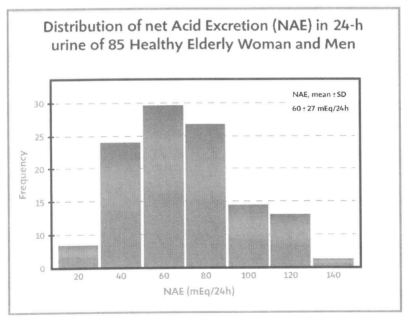

Figure 4: Distribution of net acid excretion

For some of the participants in this study, the situation was actually quite dire. Although the mean was 60 milliequivalents, a significant proportion of the participants excreted much more—in some cases above 100 milliequivalents. To excrete this much acid places the kidneys under extreme stress. Yet, if we extrapolate the findings of this study to Western civilisation as a whole, such a level of acid ingestion is an everyday reality for something like 15-20% of the population!

A complicating factor is that the older we get, the more we tend to prefer an acidic diet. A study conducted by the German Institute for Child Nutrition, in collaboration with us, compared young children, teens, young adults, and the elderly. It revealed the extent to which increased age causes us to crave a more acidic diet—at the very time when our acid excretion capacity is diminishing (Berkemeyer et al., 2008). Young children have a relatively high ability to eliminate acid. But even as teenagers, we experience a significant drop-off. By the time we are elderly, we have a severely reduced capacity. So simply by ageing, we slide into a state of acidosis.

What effect does acidosis have on our metabolism and our system in general?

Since the acid-base balance is so crucial, other parts of the body are called upon to assist with acid buffereing, mainly the bones, the connective tissues, and the intracellular aspects of the cells. Acidosis has a potent negative effect on these parts of our body and our overall wellbeing, as the body calls up its "backup systems" to keep our pH in a state of homeostasis.

We'll first zero in on the effect to the bones, for the simple reason that until recently this is where most of the research has been focused. Our area of expertise some time ago was mainly that of the metabolism of minerals. When you are interested in, for instance, the metabolism of calcium and magnesium, you are only one step from considering the body's acid-base balance. So to take this step was quite natural.

Having said this, we need to confess that as recently as twenty years ago we were somewhat sceptical that the acid-base balance of the body had any significant impact on health. Our scepticism originated from ignorance, because little research had been done in this field. During the course of the past two decades, many studies have been conducted, and they show overwhelmingly that the acid-base relationship is crucial to health. This is particularly true of the large number of studies of bone.

When we began researching in this field, we were surprised to learn that as far back as the 1960s, it was already known that acid load decreases the buffering capacity of blood. It was also understood that this decrease in buffering capacity leads to a release of minerals from the bones, which in turn significantly increases the occurrence of osteoporosis. The information was published in 1966 (Lemann et al., 1966), and again in 1968 (Wachman and Bernstein), in such highly regarded journals as The Lancet.

Unfortunately, the findings outlined in these papers failed to gain entrance into the standard medical textbooks. Consequently, in time the information was simply forgotten. The failure of this valuable information to garner the attention of the journals that it deserved wasn't the result of neglect, and neither was it suppressed for some intentional reason. Rather, the primary reason it failed to take centre stage was that determination of the acid-base ratio is an extremely complicated process, since there isn't a straightforward diagnostic tool to tell us the status of a patient's acid-base balance.

Osteoporosis has emerged as one of the great scourges of our time. The discomfort, and often disability, it causes is not only distressing but also extremely costly. Tripping up and falling over are natural occurrences that happen to us from the day we first push ourselves up off the floor, exchanging standing and walking for crawling. Most of the time, falling does little or no harm. However, in old age, because of osteoporosis, a fall can spell disaster. No one wants to fall and find themselves faced with expensive surgery and months of convalescence. If the osteoporosis is severe enough, a hip fracture can signal the end, triggering a downward slide into morbidity and death.

We don't have current data on the rate of osteoporosis in the global population. What we have is over a decade old (Frassetto et al., 2000). Nevertheless, examining the data is revelatory. Professor Vormann is German, so it distresses him to see that Germans hold the world record when it comes to the occurrence of osteoporosis. Norway, Sweden, Denmark, Argentina, New Zealand, and Switzerland are runners up.

Hip fracture rate in different countries

Country	Hip fracture rate per 100.000 years	Country	Hip fracture rate per 100.000 years
Nigeria	1	Ireland	76
China	3	France	77
New Guinea	3	Finland	94
Thailand	5	Canada	110
South Africa	8	Crete	113
Korea	11	UK	116
Singapore	22	Portugal	119
Malaysia	27	USA	120
Jugoslavia	33	Australia	124
Saudi Arabia	47	Switzerland	130
Chile	56	New Zealand	139
Italy	57	Argentina	147
Netherlands	60	Denmark	165
Spain	65	Sweden	172
Japan	67	Norway	187
Hong Kong	69	Germany	199
Israel	75		

Figure 5: Hip fracture rate across the globe

We measure hip fracture rate per 100,000 cumulative years. That is, we take a population and add their ages until they total 100,000. Then we scale the number in that population who suffer fractures. Germany comes in at 199 on the scale.

14

You may be surprised to hear us say this is no surprise. If you look at the latitude of the nations with the highest rates of osteoporosis, you will see that they all suffer a reduced intake of vitamin D from a lack of sun exposure because of their proximity to the poles—the Scandinavian countries along with Germany in the northern hemisphere, and New Zealand in the southern hemisphere. It's a well-documented fact that those countries which receive considerably less sunlight have the greatest occurrence of osteoporosis.

While this is no surprise, given our understanding of the role of vitamin D in protecting against osteoporosis, the data does nevertheless include a surprise—next on the scale is Australia at 124! A continent the world thinks of as having endless sunshine. The United States is also high at 120.

We could suggest that if you don't want to suffer from osteoporosis, you should simply move to Nigeria. There, the hip fracture rate is only one in 100,000 years! China would be a good choice also, since its rate is a mere three per 100,000 years.

What this means, of course, is that while vitamin D deficiency is an important contributor to osteoporosis, the main cause—or perhaps we should say the predisposing factor—lies elsewhere.

[4]

On the Trail
of the Causes of Osteoporosis

Upon learning that a lack of vitamin D can't be the primary factor driving the increase of osteoporosis in Western civilisation, you might be tempted to conclude that it's lack of calcium, and so we need to drink more milk, and probably also take calcium supplements. Millions in Western societies have bought into this dogma for decades.

Contrary to what you have no doubt heard in the popular press, and perhaps from your misinformed doctor, osteoporosis isn't the result of low calcium intake—and it certainly isn't caused by a milk deficiency. There's simply not a shred of evidence for what has become lore. On the other hand, there is mounting evidence that getting too much calcium in supplemental form is probably contributing to heart attacks.

We mentioned earlier that dieting to encourage weight loss imposes a significant negative effect on the acid-base balance. A study in which people fasted for four days looked at their calcium excretion (Grinspoon et al., 1995). In the control group, fasting nearly doubled the rate of calcium excretion via their urine. However, if we supplement with alkaline substances, this rapid excretion of calcium is avoided. This leads us to the conclusion that the acid-base balance significantly influences calcium loss.

In another, more sophisticated study with three phases, the subjects ingested a diet that contained relatively low protein content

(Lutz, 1984). That's quite in contrast to the diet of many so-called civilised nations. For instance, in Germany the average protein intake is around 100 to110 grams per day. In countries like Australia and the United States, it's even higher, in part as a result of the large quantities of beef these nations consume.

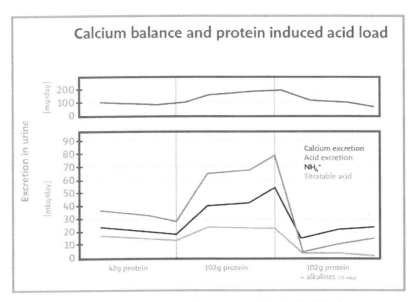

Figure 6: Calcium imbalance and protein induced acid load

When we say that the study involved a relatively low protein content, we are talking about 42 grams per day during the first phase. So this was considerably less than half what most Westerners consume in a day. The findings of this study were, to say the least, interesting. In a 24-hour urine collection, the acid excretion parameters were remarkably low, consisting of mainly ammonium ions, free acid, and titratable acid. Calcium excretion was also relatively stable.

In the second phase of the study, the quantity of protein in the diet was modified upwards, though nothing else in the individuals' lifestyles changed. This increase in daily protein intake induced an acid load, the consequence of which was almost a doubling of the level of calcium excretion.

Let us be quick to point out that during both these phases of the study, the calcium content of the diet, as well as the percentage of calcium absorbed from the diet, was identical. In other words, this is all about calcium loss. Where does the calcium come from? The bones! In fact, some 99.9% of our calcium is localised in the bones, which are our only means of storing this mineral. Do you begin to understand the connection with osteoporosis?

In the third phase of this illuminating study, participants ingested a typical high protein diet—except that to this diet were added alkaline minerals. This resulted in a neutralisation of the acid load, together with a normalisation of calcium excretion. This means that without any change in calcium intake or absorption, there is a significant effect on the human body's calcium balance simply as a result of changing the acid-base parameters.

Our conclusion to this carefully conducted study is that a state of acidosis, due to the diet, causes a loss of calcium from the bones, as calcium is the body's only truly effective way of buffering a surplus of acid.

[5]

The Chemistry Behind Osteoporosis

Unfortunately, it's not so easy to measure effects directly at the bone. However, net calcium fluxes have been measured in isolated bone tissue relative to extracellular pH (Frick et al., 2005). With a normal pH of 7.4, there is almost no flux of calcium. But even a slight decrease to 7.3 produces a significant increase in the amount of calcium released from the bones and excreted. Additionally, better calcium uptake into the bones is achieved with a more alkaline pH. In other words, the transport of calcium either into or out of the bone is directly correlated to even relatively small changes in pH. We need to point out that this isn't just a chemical effect, whereby acid dissolves bone minerals. Let me explain how it works.

It's known that acidosis activates factors in the osteoblasts, particularly the receptor NF-kappaB ligand, produced together with TNF-alpha. When both these substances work on pro-osteoclasts, they differentiate into osteoclasts which become more active (Frick and Bushinsky, 2003). It's these more-active osteoclasts that dissolve bone mass. If an activated osteoclast migrates over the bone surface, it dissolves the calcium out of the bone. As a great number of these cells migrate over the bones over a period of years, fractures occur. In other words, a change in pH in a more-acidic direction leads to significantly increased activity of osteoclasts, degrading the bones.

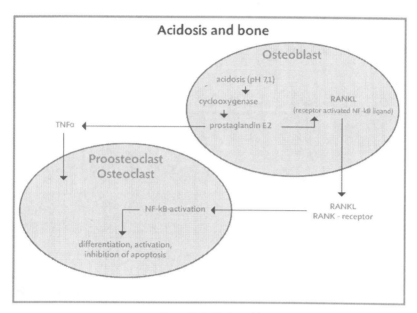

Figure 7: Acidosis and bone

Since high activity among the osteoclasts is a problem in terms of osteoporosis, to address the problem we can use pharmaceuticals to block TNFalpha and RANKL. The newest drugs actually kill the osteoclasts, which reduces the loss of bone density. The difficulty is that if we want to avoid osteoporosis by inhibiting these substances, it costs thousands of dollars a year to treat each patient, which renders the use of such pharmaceuticals as a preventive measure unviable. Thankfully, it isn't necessary to employ such costly protocols, because study after study has shown that all we have to do is avoid a state of acidosis.

For instance, a study was carried out in which the participants ingested either an acidic diet or an alkaline, base-forming diet (Buclin et al., 2001). Calcium excretion as a result of the acidic diet was shown to be much higher than the alkaline diet. Even though calcium supplements were administered to the participants in this study, they had almost zero effect on the acid-base balance, since it's much more heavily influenced by the acid-base content of the diet than by supplementation with calcium.

Another study, this time involved elderly women above the age of 75, used ultrasound to address the degree to which dietary acid load is positively associated with bone density (Wynn et al., 2008). The participants were divided into three groups. At the end of the trial, the group who received the lowest diet-induced acid burden manifested the greatest bone density.

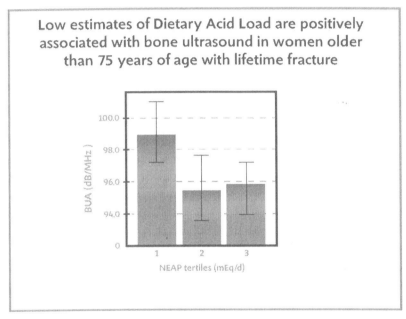

Figure 8: Dietary acid load

A similar finding emerged from a study of five groups in which bone density was measured. Using the most modern method of determining the acid load of the diet, the group with the lowest acid load came out with the greatest bone density, while there was a significant reduction of density in the group that ingested the highest acid load (Welch et al., 2007).

A large epidemiological study of 1,056 premenopausal or perimenopausal women, aged between 45 and 54, showed the same effect (New et al., 2004). Quite simply, the lower the acidity of the diet, the greater the density of the bone as measured in both the femur and the spine.

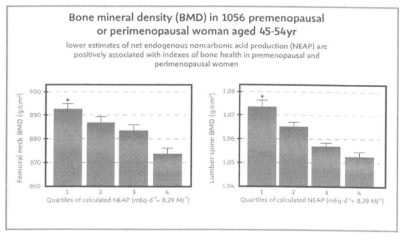

Figure 9: Bone mineral density

Additionally, in a significant number of children the diet is so acid-laden that the acid-excretion capacity of their kidneys is borderline. This was also the finding of a research group at the German Institute for Child Nutrition (Alexy et al., 2005). Their findings are in line with the view that unfavourable effects on bone health may already emerge in childhood if high endogenous acid loads aren't appropriately counterbalanced.

So what is it about alkalinity that makes the difference?

|6|

Understanding Alkalinity

When we eat an apple, it improves the acid-base ratio because of its alkaline nature. This alkalinity is mainly the result of the presence of citrates.

In a study of two groups, one of which was treated and the other of which acted as a control group, it was shown that we can reduce the acid load simply by ingesting an a supplement (Marangella et al., 2004). In this particular study, a 24-hour urine test revealed a reduction from 52 mmol down to 31 mmol, simply from taking a citrate supplement. Parameters of bone degradation—hydroxyproline and crosslinks—were also significantly reduced.

Bone metabolism and citrate supplementation
postmenopausal women, 0,1g citrate/kg b.w. daily for 3 months

Analyte	Treated N=30			Control group N=24		
	Before treatment	After followup	P	Baseline	After followup	P
pH	6.11 ± 0.68	6.33 ± 0.56	N.S.	6.13 ± 0.62	6.09 ± 0.46	N.S.
Sodium (mEq/24 hours)	108 ± 52	146 ± 53	N.S.	147 ± 49	136 ± 53	N.S.
Potassium (mEq/24 hours)	55.7 ± 38.7	79.1 ± 40.4	0.009	57.1 ± 22.2	61.9 ± 17.6	N.S.
Calcium (mg/24 hours)	162 ± 85	173 ± 98	N.S.	150 ± 44	152 ± 76	N.S.
Phosphorus (mmol/24 hours	19.4 ± 7.7	17.4 ± 5.2	N.S.	16.1 ± 4.4	16.7 ± 6.6	N.S.
Citrate (mmol/24 hours)	2.91 ± 1.63	3.84 ± 1.62	0.017	3.02 ± 1.69	2.74 ± 1.51	N.S.
Inorganic sulfate (mmol/24 hours)	15.2 ± 7.2	15.6 ± 5.3	N.S.	13.2 ± 3.9	13.3 ± 3.3	N.S.
Net acid excretion (mmol/24 hours)	52.6 ± 13.3	31.3 ± 12.9	0.004	41.4 ± 21.6	41.8 ± 21.8	N.S.
Total nitrogen excretion (mmol/24 hours)	828 ± 270	732 ± 183	N.S.	691 ± 273	691 ± 213	N.S.
Calcium (mg/mg uCr (fasting urine))	0.168 ± 0.32	0.141 ± 0.07	N.S.	0.12 ± 0.08	0.12 ± 0.09	N.S.
Hydroxyproline (mg/g uCr (fasting urine))	23.9 ± 9.1	15.3 ± 6.7	0.004	21.7 ± 7.1	19.3 ± 7.5	N.S.
Crosslinks (nmo/nmol uCr (fasting urine))	9.08 ± 2.7	7.01 ± 2.2	0.007	6.3 ± 1.7	7.3 ± 3.0	N.S.

Means ± SD are shown; P values were calculated by paired Student's t-test

Figure 10: Bone metabolism and citrate supplementation

Another yearlong study looked at 160 postmenopausal women of around 58 years of age who were suffering from osteopenia, which was already reducing their bone density (Jehle et al., 2004). Each received 30 mmol per day of either potassium chloride or potassium citrate for twelve months. We should point out that potassium chloride is a neutral salt, whereas potassium citrate is alkaline. Additionally, all 160 women received 500 milligrams of calcium and 400 IU of vitamin D.

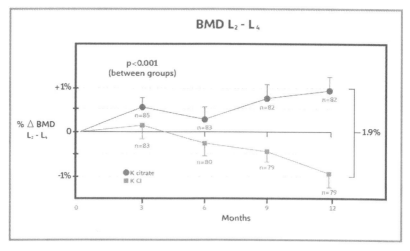

Figure 11: BMD levels

At the conclusion of the trial, even though all the women received calcium and vitamin D, which are generally thought to benefit the bones, the women who were given potassium chloride still experienced a bone density loss of about 1%—a significant and unfortunately medically relevant amount, as this is the usual loss of elderly persons sliding into osteoporosis. In contrast, the group that received potassium citrate not only avoided a decrease in bone density, but actually increased their bone density—so much so that, at the end of the year, the two groups differed by as much as 1.9%.

Interestingly, when we give a patient bisphosphonate, which is a standard treatment for osteoporosis, we get a similar response of between 1% and 2%. The downside is that there can be multiple side effects. By providing sufficient alkalinity, we can achieve the same effect as achieved by the most modern treatment for osteoporosis, minus the side effects!

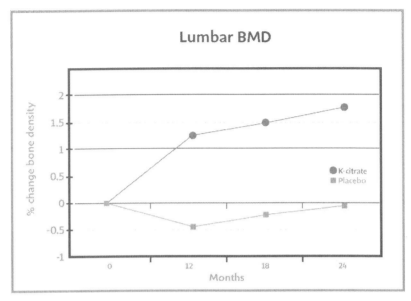

Figure 12: Lumbar BMD

Another study, from a team from Basel, Switzerland, involved 201 subjects who weren't osteopenic but were simply older (69.1 +/- 3.3 years) (Jehle et al., 2013). These were people with a normal baseline mineral density. In the randomised trial, they received either 60 mmol of potassium citrate daily or a placebo over the course of two years.

When we looked at the lumbar BMD, the placebo had pretty much no effect, whereas the potassium citrate group had a gain of nearly 2%, which is highly significant. The same was the case with hip bone density and the radius. A more complex radius measurement was also made with computer tomography, again with similar results. Further analysis of this study could show that the lifetime fracture risk was increased in the placebo group, but significantly reduced in the group taking citrate.

[7]

The Role of Protein

We mentioned earlier that people who hear this information might be tempted to simply eat less protein, since protein is acid-forming. But as another study makes clear, this isn't a good idea because protein has a positive effect on the bone mineral density. Indeed, amino acids are needed for bone building.

However, it depends on what kind of protein you eat, since the acidic content of proteins consists of the sulfur-containing amino acids. The study we referred to earlier demonstrated that a positive association of lumbar spine bone mineral density seen with dietary protein, is suppressed by a negative association with the sulfur in proteins.

If we consider soy, this is a protein that's relatively low in sulfur, so it doesn't have a negative effect in terms of the bone mineral density. (However, soy must be fermented to be healthy.) In contrast, even if we ingest low amounts of proteins, but they have a high sulfur content, there is a negative effect on bone density.

Again, we see that it's the acidity of the protein that's the deciding factor. This leads us to conclude that we should consume protein, but also a lot of alkaline food, or take alkaline supplements, in order to avoid the negative effects of acidosis. It's also important to mention that acidosis depresses protein synthesis, while simultaneously stimulating protein breakdown from skeletal muscle by activating the adenosine-triphosphate-dependent pathway involving ubiquitin and proteasomes (as reported by May et al., as far back as 1986).

A study was conducted to assess the influence of a low carbohydrate diet, such as the Atkins Diet, on the acid-base balance (Reddy et al., 2002). As you might expect, given the large amount of protein involved with the Atkins diet, adhering to this diet resulted in a significant acid burden. In fact, the level of acid excretion almost doubled. The study revealed that such a diet also has a significant effect on calcium excretion, since the acidity simply washes calcium out of the body—something that occurs even when calcium supplementation is given. Further, on Atkins-type diets, bone building is also reduced. Consequently, if you adhere to a low carbohydrate, high protein diet, which is not a bad idea with regard to reducing body weight and the risk of diabetes, it's essential to use alkaline supplementation to neutralise the effect of the sulfur.

An excessive acid load also inhibits the metabolism of fat. Yet people go on the Atkins diet precisely because they want to lose fat. This sets up a conflicting situation in the body—one that overall takes a toll on the bones. Allow us to explain why.

The high acid load of Atkins-type diets leads to loss of nitrogen. However, nitrogen is something we need in order to excrete acid. It's now well known that since we don't have a single means of storing nitrogen, the nitrogen required to excrete an excess of acid is drawn from skeletal muscle. As we age, this contributes to a loss of muscle mass. However, the good news is that the loss of nitrogen is also reduced with the use of alkaline minerals.

In summary, when there is a small change in blood pH—one that's almost undetectable—there's a concomitant change in bicarbonate and acid load that results in calcium release, a decrease in bone building activity, and accelerated bone degradation. Over the long term, this contributes significantly to osteoporosis.

We mentioned earlier that as we age, we slide into a state of acidosis. In an acidic state, we use up nitrogen from muscle. Now we begin having problems with sarcopenia, which is a degenerative loss of skeletal muscle mass. Further, although relatively small, we experience a change in our free acid secretion. Most of the acid is excreted in urine as an ammonium ion. In addition, we have more phosphate in our urine, as phosphorus is released from bone as it degenerates. It's not a pretty picture, and you can see the effects in so many older people as they appear increasingly frail, often stooped, and withered.

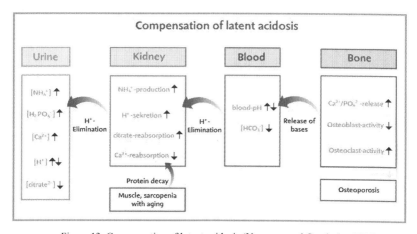

Figure 13: Compensation of latent acidosis (Vormann and Goedecke, 2006)

One more thing we should mention is that in this downward spiral, we also have less citrate, because citrate is reabsorbed in the kidneys, and as we have noted the efficiency of the kidneys declines as a result of acidosis. Less citrate also induces a significantly increased risk of kidney stones, which is one of the reasons almost 10% of the global population suffers from them. Indeed, Michael Wiederkehr and Reto Krapf report in Swiss Med Weekly (2001) that "a large proportion of renal stone formers ingesting a high protein diet have decreased urinary citrate excretion, possibly due to the diet-induced acid load." They add, "Metabolic acidosis induces a negative calcium balance (resorption from bone) with hypercalciuria and a propensity to develop kidney stones."

We hasten to say that all of this can be avoided with reasonable alkaline supplementation.

[8]

A Study Tells the Story

Generally, many doctors doubt that a problem concerning acid-base balance exists, as the blood pH is always kept constant. However, the question is whether this is also the case in the extracellular phase of the connective and other tissues. This part of the body is not readily accessible to pH measurement—and in the minds of many scientists, what you can't measure doesn't exist. But there is proof that an extracellular acidosis occurs regularly.

Elegant methods are now available to show the change in extracellular pH. For this, a study of extracellular acidosis involved six subjects (Street et al., 2001). The idea was to determine the interstitial pH in calf muscle of several subjects after five minutes of working out on an exercise bicycle with an ergometer, utilising workloads of 30, 50, and 70 watts. This isn't a particularly difficult level of exercise, and any one of us could do it easily.

In this study, using a highly complicated procedure, the muscle was perfused with a pH-sensitive dye. The pH-dependent change in the dye was detected in vivo (within)—a somewhat unpleasant process. This means it isn't a test we can run with regular patients. Thankfully, some students were willing to suffer a little for a good cause!

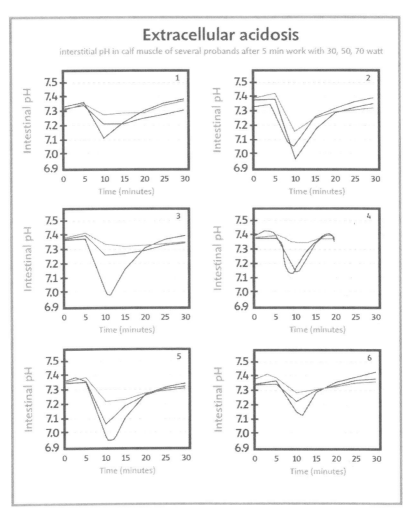

Figure 14: Extracellular acidosis—interstitial pH in calf muscle

The candidates all began with a textbook 7.4 pH. After only five minutes' workload, the pH dropped significantly—even below 7.0. After stopping the exercise, it took about twenty minutes for full recovery of the pH to occur. This was the first study to demonstrate that extracellular acidosis is a state that truly exists, at least locally and for a certain period. Each of the six candidates had a different response, perhaps connected with their level of physical training, along with their diet.

A second study used the same basic methodology. This time pH was shown as the acid concentration, meaning the concentration of protons was directly depicted (Street et al., 2005). One group of students was given a placebo, whereas the other group received alkaline supplementation. The alkaline supplementation successfully suppressed the increased acidity that resulted from working out with the ergometer. If we think back to our evolution as a species, hunters-gatherers moved a lot more than most of us do today, both walking and, for short bursts, running. However, they ingested a highly alkaline diet, thereby avoiding the negative effects of the workload on their extracellular pH.

We need to point out that as the pH changes when we take on a workload, it quickly becomes high enough to activate the osteoclasts of cells. In other words, a relatively normal workload activates bone degradation for perhaps half an hour or so. While the effect isn't dramatic, over a period of years it adds up. We can avoid such negative effects if we have sufficient buffering capacity in our connective tissues.

If we look at the structure of our connective tissues, one has to distinguish between the intracellular space and extracellular space. In the extracellular space, molecules of collagen, which is a group of proteins found especially in the connective tissues, are accompanied by feather-like structures generally referred to as aminoglycans or proteoglycans. These fulfil an important function, in that they carry a high negative charge, involving millions upon millions of negatively charged particles. This negative charge is needed to bind water in the connective tissues, a process that's extremely important for our physiological functioning.

We can illustrate what happens by asking you to stand on one leg. Do you feel the pressure on the cartilage in your knee? Part of this pressure is absorbed by the fact that some of the water is squeezed out of the cartilage. Then, when the pressure is released, the water flows back into the cartilage. This physical buffering system only works because of water binding. The ability of the body to bind water is also necessary for many other functions, not least of which is the transport of nutrients to the various cells.

What happens when we experience local acidosis? Imagine more and more acid in the area of your knee. The acid neutralises the negative charge, reducing the overall water binding capacity of your connective tissues. As your water binding capacity decreases, it leads to a loss of elasticity, contributing to the impairment of cartilage, tendons, and ligaments. The result is increased rigidity. This process continues on a routine basis in so many of us, leading to joint problems.

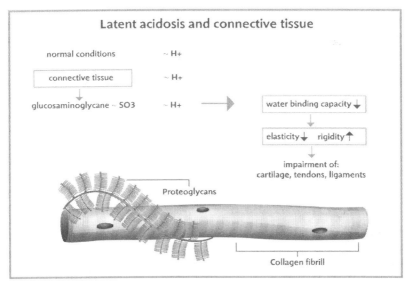

Figure 15: Latent acidosis and connective tissue

[9]

A Different Understanding
of Chronic Pain

One of the most debilitating forms of chronic pain occurs in the lower back. Thankfully, we can offer you some hope if you suffer from this.

Some years ago we did an observational study that, in addition to their usual medication, treated patients suffering from chronic low back pain were treated with alkalising minerals over the course of a four-week period (Vormann et al., 2001). We quantified their pain using the Arhus low back pain rating scale, which is a validated method of determining a patient's status. It consists of a questionnaire concerning back and leg pain, use of analgesics, the degree of disability, and so on. When we administered the questionnaire again at the end of the month's trial, we learned that simply by supplementing with alkaline minerals, we were able to reduce patients' pain by more than 50%. Disability and physical impairment were also reduced. Please note that these were all patients who were using pain medication regularly because of their chronic back problems.

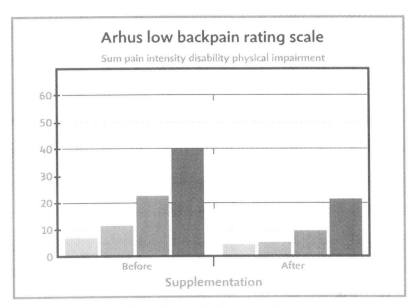

Figure 16: Arhus low back pain rating scale

The wonderful thing about alkalising minerals is that they provide us with an alternative treatment that doesn't have side effects. Since the patients' pain was so greatly reduced, it meant that their use of analgesics could also be lowered. Patients with this kind of pain tend to take a lot of medication to manage their pain, which over the long-term can have significant side effects. The reduction of such medication is a tremendous blessing.

Alkalising Minerals and low back pain

The intake of Alkalising Minerals reduced pain symptoms in patients with chronic low back pain by more than 50%.

The use of analgesics could be reduced.

Physical impairment was improved.

Alkalising Minerals is an alternative without side effects for chronic low back pain caused by a disturbed acid-base homeostasis.

The study also gave us a hint that chronic low back pain may even be caused by a disturbed acid-base homeostasis. When glucosaminoglycans are more neutralised, the body's capacity for water binding decreases.

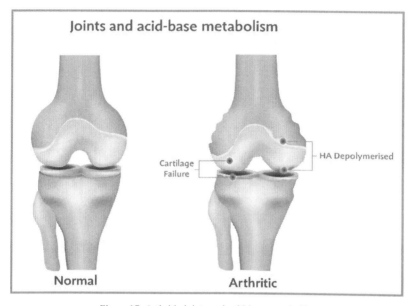

Figure 17: Arthritic joints and acid-base metabolism

There is some evidence that rheumatoid arthritis may also be influenced by changes in the connective tissue, occasioned by reduced water binding. If we look at a normal versus an arthritic joint, it has been shown that the synovial fluid in the joint is significantly more acidic (Farr et al., 1985).

This is because the inflammation in the cartilage produces acid. In patients with rheumatoid arthritis, the acid load in the knee joint is much higher than in patients with osteoarthritis or other forms of arthritis.

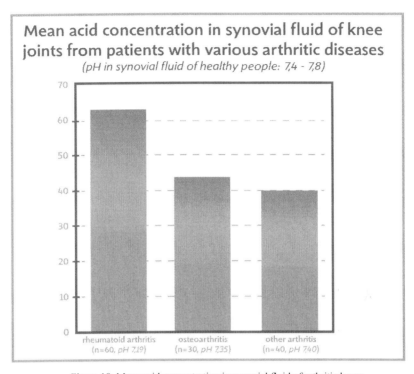

Figure 18: Mean acid concentration in synovial fluid of arthritic knees

Unfortunately, this study omitted to measure healthy controls. It's not easy to convince healthy people to allow us to punctuate the knee joint and measure their pH—a quite unpleasant experience. From other studies, it's known that the pH of the synovial fluid in patients suffering from rheumatoid arthritis is around 25 nmol H^+/l. What is the effect of this increased acidity? Certainly, there is the effect of painful arthritic joints. But is this just an effect of disturbed extracellular water binding, or might it be that a change in acidity influences pain sensation directly?

Again using students, a study conducted in Japan was designed to investigate small pH changes for their impact on pain (Ugawa et al., 2002). The students were subcutaneously injected with a saline solution of varying pH levels. Remember the earlier comment regarding dipping your finger into concentrated hydrochloric acid—

we would only ever do it once! Concentrated acid has a pH of 1 or 2, so the burning effect is excruciating. In this study, not surprisingly, small changes in pH significantly increased the sensation of pain, with zero on the scale representing no pain and 10 representing the most intense agony a person can imagine. The astonishing thing is that these students were driven into the most extreme pain—a level so extreme that no ethical committee in Germany, Australia, or the U.S. would have allowed the study there.

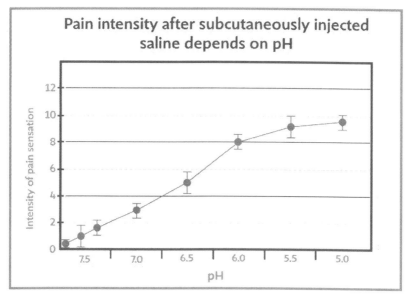

Figure 19: Pain intensity

Amazingly, a small change in fluid pH from 7.4 to 7.0 significantly increases the sensation of pain. Remember that this change in pH may happen in the extracellular space of our muscles when we are exercising intensely.

What is the mechanism behind this sensitivity to acid? Is it just an acid-induced destroying of biological structures?

In recent years, it has been determined that humans have a large number of pain receptors in their nerves that react to acid (Holzer,

2009). For instance, our ion channel subunits and receptors are modulated by extracellular acid. The cell membrane has receptors, among which the acid-sensing ion channels are especially important. At a pH of 7.4, the channels are usually closed, meaning there's no pain. These are sodium channels, so when they are closed, sodium can't pass through them. When we have an increasing quantity of extracellular acid, this acid binds to these channels, inducing a change in structure that causes them to open. Then sodium enters the cell, resulting in the nerve sending a signal of "pain" to the brain.

From a pharmacological point of view, this system is so intriguing that many groups worldwide are investigating whether there are substances that can block these channels. If we can block them, we have a pain medication. (If you are the first to do it, you will unquestionably become a billionaire since so many people on the planet suffer with this kind of pain!) What we are anxious to get across to you is that we can achieve the same effect far more easily by supplying sufficient alkaline to perform effective buffering. In this way, we prevent the pH in this localised area from become low enough to cause the channels to open. Alkaline supplementation is therefore automatically pain medication!

Professor Vormann collaborated on a study of patients who were being treated in a specialty clinic in Budapest, Hungary, for chronic rheumatoid arthritis (Cseuz et al., 2008). In addition to the standard therapy, the candidates were supplemented for twelve weeks with a daily dosage of 30 grams of an alkalising mineral supplement. If we look at the results on a disease-associated symptom index, this index fell significantly in those who received the supplements. We also observe that the reduction of pain after four weeks was significant, and by eight weeks had fallen almost 50%. In contrast, pain increased in the control group.

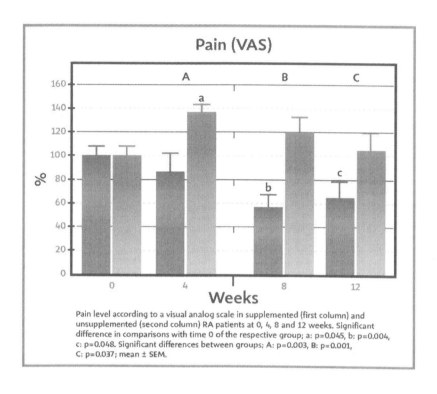

Pain level according to a visual analog scale in supplemented (first column) and unsupplemented (second column) RA patients at 0, 4, 8 and 12 weeks. Significant difference in comparisons with time 0 of the respective group; a: p=0.045, b: p=0.004, c: p=0.048. Significant differences between groups; A: p=0.003, B: p=0.001, C: p=0.037; mean ± SEM.

Figure 20: Pain (VAS)

Also, in terms of the physical functioning of the patients, the reduction seen in the treated group represents an improvement. Other pain medications simply can't match the effects achieved in this study.

However, this study showed us that we must be patient when we use alkaline supplementation. We can't expect it to work within hours like analgesics. It takes some time for the alkalinity to flood the system, penetrating the tissues, joints, and so forth. We have determined that a program of alkaline supplementation requires at least four weeks before there's a significant effect. At eight weeks, the effect is considerably greater, at twelve weeks it's quite profound. We don't know what happens beyond the three-month mark, since we haven't yet been able to extend a study over a more prolonged period due to the cost involved. Yet many of the patients involved in the study continued to take the supplementation after the end of the trial and reported persistent improvement.

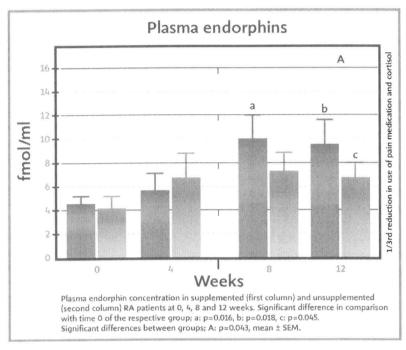

Figure 21: Plasma endorphins

The chart above represents the measurement of plasma endorphin concentration in these patients. Endorphins are our "happy" hormones and, when in adequate supply, they lead to a significant improvement in our wellbeing. In the alkaline supplemented group, the concentration of endorphins had significantly increased by eight weeks. This, combined with pain reduction and increased mobility, meant that the patients' overall sense of wellbeing was considerably improved.

Once again, a plus is that we were able to reduce pain medication and the use of cortisone by a third, which is a very beneficial effect. We don't claim that alkaline supplementation can heal rheumatoid arthritis; so far, there's only symptomatic treatment for the disease.

Nevertheless, alkaline supplementation has a truly positive benefit. Aside from improving the physical state of connective tissue and stabilisation of pain receptors, the positive effect of alkaline supplementation may also be explained by effects on the inflammatory processes.

It's now known, from a study released in 2012, that acidosis has a major pro-inflammatory effect (Etulain et al., 2012). Extracellular acidosis down-regulates platelet haemostatic functions and (in our opinion, even more important) amplifies inflammatory response. So all the inflammation going on in a person is worsened if, in addition, there is acidosis. Again, reducing the acidosis has a positive effect on the inflammation.

So the reasonable increase in alkaline mineral intake may work through multiple mechanisms, and it remains to be established which mechanism contributed most to the overall positive results.

[10]

Acidosis and Alzheimer's

When it comes to the effect of acidosis on neurological functioning, an interesting study highlights the influence of our acid-base balance on IQ. The intracellular pH in the central nervous system of 42 boys was determined and correlated with their IQ (Rae et al., 1996). The study was non-invasive. In other words, it didn't involve insertion of electrodes into the brain. The results are intriguing. How shall we put it? The more acidic, the more "stupid."

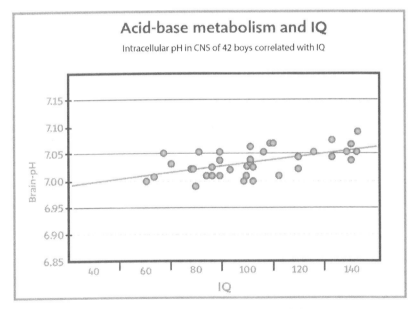

Figure 22: Acid-base metabolism and IQ

You can see from the chart that a relatively small change in pH can have a significant long-term effect on the functioning of cells.

There's a connection with Alzheimer's disease. We have biochemical evidence that a change in pH leads to aggregation of the Alzheimer's tau protein (Atwood et al., 1998). Specifically, when a normal 7.4 pH declines to a more acidic 6.8, it occasions a significant aggregation of this protein. If we then reduce the acidity, the aggregation of this protein is dissolved. Simply by changing the pH, we can determine how intensively this Alzheimer's protein is deposited. The problem, of course, is that the more this protein is deposited at the nerves, the greater the influence on the functioning of these nerves.

A recent review demonstrates this finding. Addressing the dysfunction that might cause Alzheimer's disease, it shows that both vascular damage and damage to the connective tissues leads to acidosis (Humpel, 2011). This has a deleterious effect on the metabolic function, as well as being a risk factor for the building of beta amyloid plaque (the kind of plaque associated with Alzheimer's). Many other experimental studies hint that this plaque is worsened by acidosis.

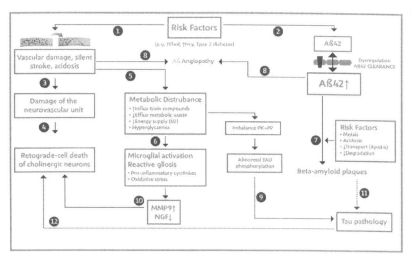

Figure 23: Risk Factors

Having said this, from a clinical point of view, it's extremely complicated to determine whether acidosis is causative or is simply one factor in the development of Alzheimer's. We would have to treat something like 20,000 people for two decades with either alkaline supplementation or a placebo, then tally how many cases of Alzheimer's occur in the two groups—a study that's simply not possible, given the cost. Despite this, we have strong chemical evidence that acidosis has something to do with this condition, especially considering its influence on the building of plaque.

In addition to the biochemical findings concerning acidosis and cognition, it's interesting to note the impressions of many users of alkaline supplements. After several days of initial use, many of them note that they feel psychologically more energised and relieved. If small amounts of protein debris have been deposited along nerves, these might be cleared in a less acidic environment, giving the nerves the chance to function better. Unfortunately, currently we don't possess the diagnostic tools to identify such deposits in our central nervous system.

[11]

The Cancer Connection

You might wonder, is there any connection between acidosis and cancer?

Many years ago now, Otto Warburg in Germany described how cancer cells produce more acid than normal cells, a discovery for which he received a Nobel Prize. Normal tissue has an extracellular pH of 7.4, whereas testing of various forms of cancer in mice, rats, and humans has shown that the extracellular pH is significantly reduced. The pain cancer patients experience is connected to the acidosis that's induced by the cancer. The pH also falls within the cells.

Cancer cells must multiply if a cancer is to thrive. To do so the cells need space, which is a problem if the area surrounding the cancer cells is densely packed with healthy cells. To combat this, the cancer cells produce acid and secrete this acid into the surrounding cells. Since these normal cells can't cope with this level of acidity over long periods of time, the acidity gradually kills them, whereupon they are broken down and excreted from the body. This creates the space for the cancer cells to replicate.

A relatively new study demonstrated the effect of increased acidity on the evolution of breast cancer over time (Robey and Martin, 2011). In the beginning we simply have a few cancer cells. But, as they generate more and more acid, destroying normal cells in the process, we end up with an invasive cancer that produces metastases.

Cell cultures have shown us that the consequences of tumour acidity are multifaceted, involving spontaneous transformation, radio resistance, hyperthermic sensitisation, ion trapping of weak base drugs, increased in vivo metastasis, more virulent invasion, increased chromosomal rearrangement, a heightened mutation rate, and altered gene expression—all of which contribute to cancer.

Consequences of tumor acidity

- Spontaneous tranformation
- Radio resistance
- Hyperthermic sensitization
- Ion trapping of weak base drugs
- Increased in vivo metastasis
- Increased invasion
- Increased mutation rate
- Increased chromosomal rearrangements
- Altered gene expression

It would be interesting to see whether, using alkaline supplementation, it might be possible to reduce the growth of cancer. There are no clinical studies in humans on this; however, a recent study involving experiments with mice began to supply some answers.

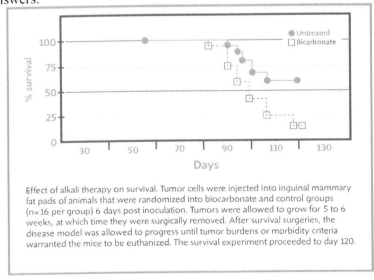

Effect of alkali therapy on survival. Tumor cells were injected into inguinal mammary fat pads of animals that were randomized into biocarbonate and control groups (n=16 per group) 6 days post inoculation. Tumors were allowed to grow for 5 to 6 weeks, at which time they were surgically removed. After survival surgeries, the disease model was allowed to progress until tumor burdens or morbidity criteria warranted the mice to be euthanized. The survival experiment proceeded to day 120.

Figure 24: Effect of alkali therapy on survival

Tumour cells were injected into inguinal mammary fat pads of mice randomised into a group that received bicarbonate and a control group six days post inoculation. In other words, the mice were either left untreated or treated with alkaline bicarbonate. Tumours were allowed to grow for five to six weeks, at which time they were surgically removed. The cancer was then allowed to progress until either the tumour burden or morbidity warranted the mice to be euthanised. The survival experiment continued to day 120, with the survival rate much higher in the treated group than in the untreated group. This is the first practical evidence that alkaline supplementation may reduce the growth of cancer.

We also have some evidence from individual patients who have experienced alkaline supplementation. From these cases, many doctors have the impression that compared to other patients, those treated with alkalising minerals experienced a slower growth of tumours. Nevertheless, so far we have no placebo-controlled study of this, since such studies are so complicated and therefore expensive, given that it would be difficult to patent an alkaline supplement and make a profit. It's challenging to find a sponsor willing to invest the sum required.

[12]

Acid-base Balance
and Metabolic Diseases

A connection between latent acidosis and metabolic diseases like type 2 diabetes was proposed by researchers at the National Institute of Health (USA) some years ago (Adeva and Souto, 2011). They described the evidence that an acidogenic diet leads to chronic metabolic acidosis that induces resistance to the action of insulin.

This insulin resistance is one of the leading factors of metabolic syndrome in diabetes and cardiovascular diseases. Epidemiological data from Japan supports this (Otsuki et al., 2011). A correlation between visceral obesity and metabolic syndrome and urinary pH was found—the more acidic the higher the risk. Another large epidemiological study in Europe investigated the connection between dietary acid intake and risk for type 2 diabetes in more than 66,000 subjects (Fagherazzi et al., 2014). A significantly increased risk with higher dietary acid-load was obvious.

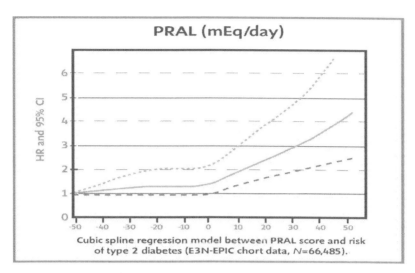

Figure 25: PRAL score and risk of diabetes

The same was found in another epidemiological study from Japan (Akter et al., 2015). The Furukawa Nutrition and Health Study reported an association between dietary acid-load and insulin resistance.

Human intervention studies done in Australia also support the notion that high dietary acid-load may contribute to insulin resistance and metabolic syndrome (Williams et al., 2015). In this study a clear correlation between the intake of alkalising minerals, especially magnesium and potassium, and disease risks was observed.

One of the main pathophysiological mechanisms for these effects of acid-base balance on metabolism is an increased release of glucocorticoid hormones esp. cortisol in latent acidosis. In the long term, this diet induced change in acid-base balance that could have a significant impact on our metabolism.

Alkaline Supplementation and Weight Loss

It is generally accepted that being overweight is a major risk factor for various diseases. Even though it is discussed whether body mass index (BMI) alone is an appropriate indicator of adiposity, the combination of BMI with measurements of body composition can reliably estimate individual health risks. Overweight individuals use numerous strategies for losing weight.

Two aspects are taken into account—increased physical activity and reduced intake of calories. To follow a calorie-restricted diet is a difficult task for the majority of overweight people. However, a general reduction of caloric intake can also be achieved by simply leaving out meals or including single days with very low intake of calories into the weekly life plan. This "intermittent fasting" has been shown to have positive and lasting effects on body weight. Also, exercise training has many proven beneficial health effects but alone is only of minor efficacy for weight reduction. Therefore, a combination of intermittent fasting with exercise training, should improve the effects of both strategies alone.

The metabolism in overweight people following an exercise program with or without caloric reduction is significantly changed into a more fat mobilising direction. As a result, a shift into a more acidic metabolic state might occur that could reduce fat metabolism. Unfortunately, this reduces the efficacy of weight loss, as a more acidic environment has been shown to reduce triglyceride metabolism and release from fat cells (Hood and Tannen. 1998). Alkaline supplementation could circumvent this effect leading to a metabolic state allowing greater weight loss.

To test this hypothesis we performed a study with overweight persons that followed an individualized exercise program for 12 weeks (Hottenrott et al., 2016). All 85 participants ingested a balanced diet. By randomization, half of the participants were assigned to follow a specific plan of integrating fasting days into their weekly routine. In addition, both groups were further split into subgroups by receiving either an alkaline mineral supplement (Basica-Direkt®) or a placebo in a randomized double-blind way.

The results of this elaborate study were very promising. Generally, intermittent fasting, in combination with the exercise program, led to a significant and meaningful weight loss. It was however remarkable that the weight loss was significantly further enhanced by taking the alkaline supplement. After 3 months of training and intermittent fasting the study participants had lost a mean 6.5 kg of body weight in the placebo group but 9.4 kg in the group taking the alkaline supplement.

Fasting, in addition to an exercise program, might induce systemic or local acidosis. Aside of interference with intracellular fat mobilisation and metabolism, the urinary excretion of ketones is reduced in acidosis by inhibiting reuptake of ketones from primary urine. Alkaline supplementation overcomes this effect, leading to a loss of energy being bound in the ketones.

The effect of the alkaline supplement on acid-base balance could be seen by an increased bicarbonate concentration in serum in the treatment groups. In addition, urinary pH was more alkaline in these groups. Even though only about 1% of total excreted acid is free and can be detected by urine-pH sticks, this change in urinary pH, together with the improved buffering capacity in serum, proves the alkaline effect of the supplement. It must be mentioned that in addition to the alkalinity, the supplement also contains minerals. Concerning serum concentration of magnesium, calcium, potassium and sodium there were no significant differences between the groups, indicating that the main effect of the supplement is due to its alkalinity.

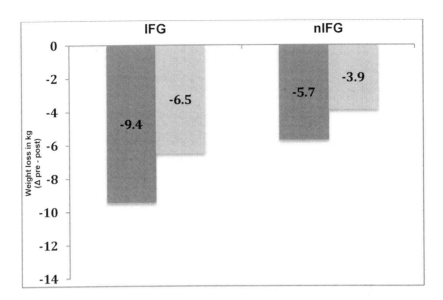

Figure 26: Weight loss of intermittent fasting group (IFG) and non-intermittent fasting group (nIFG)

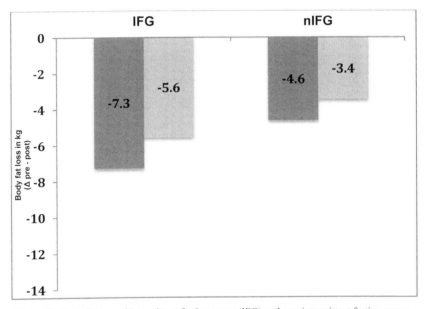

Figure 27: Body fat loss of intermittent fasting group (IFG) and non-intermittent fasting group

(nIFG)

Alkaline Supplementation and Cellular Energy Metabolism

Generally, the effect of an alkaline supplement cannot readily be seen by changes in the blood, as it is extremely buffered. However, the many positive clinical effects of alkaline supplementation allow the speculation that a more alkaline environment might have direct positive effects on cellular metabolism. As already described, small but significant changes in muscular pH can be measured after exercise. However, it was not investigated how an alkaline supplementation influences the cellular production of metabolites.

Aside from exercise, the diet might also influence the local acid-base balance. Protein-rich diets, especially, may result in chronic latent metabolic acidosis and impaired structure and function of organs, such as bone and skeletal muscle.

In a double-blind, placebo-controlled clinical trial it was tested whether a protein-rich diet given for four weeks would impair systemic and local (muscle) acid-base balance and metabolism and whether a daily supplementation with alkaline salts would prevent these changes (Boschmann et al., 2016). Forty elderly healthy men and women (60-70y, non-diabetics) were randomised to a supplemented mixture of alkaline salts (Basica-Direkt®) or placebo, and in addition they were asked to take a protein-rich diet over four weeks. The parameters were changes in systemic and skeletal muscular (M. vastus lateralis) acid-base balance by indirect calorimetry, as well as carbohydrate and lipid metabolisms by microdialysis. By this method, changes in metabolite concentrations can directly be determined in the local surrounding of the muscle cell. Measurements were done before and after intervention, both times after 12h overnight fast and after a 30g protein load within test-meals.

After four weeks, there were no significant changes for baseline systemic and local acid-base balance and metabolism in both groups. However, after the acid load of the test meal, plasma bicarbonate

54

decreased in the placebo group but not in the group taking the supplement. Plasma glucose did not change significantly in both groups. However, in the treatment group the insulin response to the test meal was significantly reduced by 9%. In the placebo group it increased by 14 %, compared to the baseline measurements, before starting the supplementation. A reduced need for insulin is a positive effect, as less need for insulin release reduces the risk for diabetes in the long term.

The metabolic state and energy supply to the muscle cells can be estimated by measuring the lactate and pyruvate concentration in the tissue. Lactate is the end product of anaerobic energy metabolism and is produced from pyruvate by the enzyme lactate dehydrogenase. This consumes the energy substrate NADH. Furthermore, pyruvate is no longer available to enter the mitochondria for oxidative metabolism. In total, this reduces the possible energy supply for the muscle. A higher pyruvate concentration on the contrary is a sign of an improved energy supply to the cell. The lactate concentration increased by about 50% in both groups after the test meal. However, the baseline level of pyruvate was only increased in the group having received the alkaline supplement.

Taken together these results show impressively, and for the first time, that alkaline supplementation improves the cellular energy supply and reduces the need for insulin. The correlation of an increased diabetes risk, with increasing acidity of the diet, could therefore be explained by the positive protective effect of a more alkaline diet.

[13]

Assessing the Effect of Diet

A review (Pizzorno et al., 2009) that was published in the prestigious British Journal of Nutrition was entitled, "Diet-induced acidosis: is it real and clinically relevant?" The authors came to the conclusion that the "available research makes a compelling case that diet-induced acidosis, not diet-induced acidaemia, is a real phenomenon, and has a significant, clinical, long-term pathophysiological effect that should be recognised and potentially counterbalanced by dietary means." The term "dietary" includes the possibility of supplementation.

Is there a way to estimate the effect of diet on acid-base metabolism?

The acid-base status of an individual can be ascertained by determining the pH of urine. However, 99% of the acid in urine isn't free acid but is in a bound form. This means that the pH sticks you can buy at a pharmacy measure only 1% of the total excretion of acid. Such a measurement may be of some value if used over a prolonged period. However, if you measure your pH just once or twice and find it's slightly acidic, it doesn't automatically mean you have acidosis. The better approach is to determine the amount of acid excreted during a 24-hour period, though for several reasons we don't find this a convenient means of gathering clinical evidence.

What we can do is estimate dietary acid load from the acid/alkaline content of food, the relative bioavailability of acid or alkaline-forming food constituents, and the potential renal acid load values of foods (PRAL).

Profs. Remer and Manz from the Research Institute for Child Nutrition in Germany, developed tables that are now widely available and used globally in epidemiological and clinical studies (Remer and Manz, 1995). The tables show the potential renal acid load of a particular food. In other words, we can identify how acidic a food is. Research comparing the analysed endogenous acid production in healthy children and juveniles with the estimates predicted by the tables, demonstrates that the values in the tables are valid.

The lower the number the more alkaline, the higher the number the more acidic. Zero is neutral.

PRAL Food List Table per 100g

Meat and Meat Products Average	9.5	Milk, Dairy, and Eggs	
Lean Beef	7.8	Milk and non-cheese average	1.0
Chicken	8.7	Low protein cheese average	8.0
Canned, Corned Beef	13.2	High protein cheese average	23.6
Frankfurters	6.7	Buttermilk	0.5
Liver Sausage	10.6	Low Fat Cheddar	26.4
Lunch Meat	10.2	Gouda Cheese	18.6
Lean Pork	7.9	Cottage Cheese	8.7
Rump Steak	8.8	Sour Cream	1.2
Salami	11.6	Whole Egg	8.2
Turkey Meat	9.9	Egg White	1.1
Veal Fillet	9.0	Egg Yolk	23.4
		Hard Cheese	19.2
Fish Average	7.9	Ice Cream	0.6
Cod Fillet	7.1	Whole milk	1.1
Haddock	6.8	Whole Milk Pasteurized	0.7
Herring	7.0	Parmesan Cheese	34.2
Trout	10.8	Processed Cheese	28.7
		Whole Milk Yogurt w/Fruit	1.2
		Whole Milk Yogurt Plain	1.5

* This table is adapted from: Remer T and Manz F. Potential renal acid load of foods and it's influence on urine pH. Journal of the American Dietetic Association. 1995.

Figure 28: PRAL food list table

Most of what we drink is alkaline, including coffee—with the exception of soft drinks. People tend to think of coffee as an acidic beverage. The discrepancy lies in the fact that there are two separate effects of drinking coffee. The first is the effect on the overall acid-base balance. The second is the effect on acid production in the stomach. Coffee might induce the production of hydrochloric acid in the stomach, although overall it's more alkaline in terms of its effect on the metabolism. In other words, for reasons explained in a moment, the production of acid in the stomach has no overall effect on the body's overall acid-base balance.

The problem with sodas or soft drinks is their phosphate content. If you drink a litre, you are getting a lot of phosphates. In contrast, you could compensate for your acidosis by simply drinking several litres of beer every day, since beer is alkaline. Of course, you would soon have other problems!

Fish and seafood are on the acidic side because they contain a high dose of protein. In contrast, all vegetables, salads, and most fruit are on the alkaline side. However, all forms of cereal, flour, bread, and pastries are on the acidic side. So if you eat a large steak together with a large portion of noodles such as spaghetti, you have a high intake of acid, since both kinds of food are extremely acid-forming. And, of course, you will have no space left in your stomach for the kind of foods that would provide you with neutralising alkalinity, such as vegetables. Here you see one of the main reasons so many in the Western world have an acid load. Especially in Germany, as they eat a lot of bread with their proteins.

It's important to be aware that while all vegetables are alkaline, 100 grams of vegetables is less alkaline than 100 grams of meat is acidic. This means that if you eat a large steak, it's not enough to eat a tomato with it to compensate for the acid load. For every 100 grams of meat, it's necessary to eat about 400 grams of vegetables or salad, which isn't something most people do. The typical dinner salad consisting of mostly lettuce that accompanies a steak dinner in a restaurant simply doesn't cut it.

Meat and meat products, such as sausages, as well as eggs, milk, and other dairy products, are on the acidic side. Given that this is the case, how much sense does it make to tell people with osteoporosis to eat plenty of cheese and drink lots of milk, which has been standard medical advice for a long time now? By the way, parmesan cheese is the world champion in terms of acid load, whereas whey is the one dairy product that's alkalising.

What we cannot say is that foodstuffs that are acidic are bad and not to be eaten, whereas those that are alkaline-forming are good and to be ingested freely. Even though it's a highly concentrated protein, you can eat parmesan cheese. But if you eat it, you need to eat it with foodstuffs that are alkaline, such as a large portion of vegetables or salad. Grated onto salad, it provides a flavourful accent. Herbs, such as basil and parsley, can also be included to add flavour, since they are especially alkalinising.

When it comes to sweets, you may be surprised to hear that white sugar is absolutely neutral. On the other hand, if you eat a sugar-rich diet, you'll have problems with acid production in the stomach. But again, this has no effect on the acid-base balance. If you look at the tables, some sweets such as honey and marmalade (which contains alkaline fruits) are alkaline, whereas others such as madeira cake are acidic.

[14]

Are Your Adrenals at Risk? How an Alkaline Diet May Help

We have talked a great deal about bone loss in conjunction with an acid-loaded diet. We want to turn now to a spinoff from the studies in this field. Research looking into latent acidosis and bone demineralisation has found that one of the ways acidosis leads to bone loss involves an increase in glucocorticoid production. It turns out that an underlying endocrine involvement has far-reaching implications in terms of the adrenals, stress hormones such as cortisol, and even thyroid hormone production.

A study that appeared in the American Journal of Renal Physiology found that latent acidosis causes a hyper-glucocorticoid response (Maurer et al., 2003). An acid-loaded diet was found to trigger increases in cortisol secretion and plasma concentrations of cortisol. In contrast, the neutralisation of the dietary acid load resulted in significant reductions in cortisol secretions, plasma concentrations of cortisol and its metabolites, and an overall drop in urinary cortisol. In this report   Maurer and colleagues states categorically, "An acidogenic Western diet results in mild metabolic acidosis in association with a state of cortisol excess, altered divalent ion metabolism, and increased bone resorptive indices." The report adds that their results "furnish the first evidence that a very mild Western diet-induced" state of acidosis, which they describe as "a degree of acidosis that would not be recognised by applying diagnostic acid-base criteria found in textbooks," results in a state of increased cortisol secretion and plasma concentration. As we have been seeing, it doesn't take much of a change in pH to cause havoc with the bones. Now we also know that the effect of even mild acidosis is far more all-encompassing than its role in osteoporosis.

Today, there is much discussion among the more health conscious concerning adrenal exhaustion. More and more alternative health practitioners are recognising how widespread adrenal fatigue is today. Symptoms of adrenal fatigue are abundantly described on a variety of internet sites, with quizzes to help the reader detect if they may be suffering from this condition. It's being blamed for such conditions as asthma, bronchitis, the common cough, allergies, muscle weakness, back pain, disturbed sleep, haemorrhoids, varicose veins, indigestion, hypoglycaemia, constipation, low self-esteem, lowered resistance to inflection, headaches, and so on.

The condition of adrenal fatigue is often said to be linked, among other factors, to improper functioning of the thyroid, as well as to either acute or prolonged stress. According to a review (Wiederkehr and Krapf, 2001), "Chronic metabolic acidosis in humans slightly decreases free T3 and free T4 and significantly increases TSH serum concentrations with no change in reverse T3, findings consistent with a primary decrease in thyroid hormone secretion, i.e. mild primary hypothyroidism." This is another indication of the role acidosis plays in a variety of ills.

The adrenal glands supply us with the ability to respond to stressful situations, equipping us for either "fight or flight". As such, they have a lot to do with why so many of us, in our stressed-out society, are continuously anxious, since so much of modern life is far from relaxed but keeps us in a state of high alert. It's known that while cortisol is essential for handling stress, prolonged stress results in negative effects, such as blood sugar imbalances, increased abdominal fat, impaired cognitive performance, increased risk of depression, suppressed thyroid function, decreased bone density, a decrease in muscle, elevated blood pressure, and lowered immunity.

Several studies have investigated whether cortisol production, and hence the adrenal glands, are affected by ingesting the higher dietary protein levels many of us in Western society consume. As an example of such studies, Maurer and colleagues looked at serum levels of cortisol and urinary excretion of total cortisol metabolites when sodium and potassium chloride were replaced by sodium and potassium bicarbonate, both of which have an acid buffering effect, in a normal diet. The excretion of cortisol and the major cortisol metabolites proved to be significantly lower under the alkalinising impact of the bicarbonates. (As explained elsewhere, other studies show that citrates are preferable to bicarbonates.)

Mark F. McCarty comments in the journal Medical Hypotheses (2005) that "there is much previous evidence that chronic metabolic acidosis is associated with increased glucocorticoid production." He adds, "The physiological trigger for this induction of glutaminase appears to be an increased adrenal production of both cortisol and aldosterone..." We have little doubt that individuals suffering from extreme anxiety, including PTSD and even suicidal tendencies driven by depression and anxiety, would benefit from correcting their overly acidic state.

The article goes on to report that Maurer's findings suggest a more subtle effect may be evoked by normal dietary conditions that provoke mild systemic acidosis, citing "a high-protein diet relatively poor in potassium-rich fruits and vegetables" as problematic. The article comments that the acidifying impact of protein reflects the fact that methionine and cysteine are metabolised to yield free sulfuric acid, whereas organic anions present in food that "yield bicarbonate when metabolized—for e.g., citrate—have a countervailing alkalinizing impact..." We have already noted the connection to sulfur.

It further states that "a diet which promotes an acidic metabolic environment will tend to promote visceral obesity and insulin resistance syndrome via a modest up-regulation of cortisol production—whereas diets promoting a more alkaline metabolic environment may be protective in this regard." While a diet high in protein helps with appetite control, thus improving insulin sensitivity, the article further states, that "conceivably it would be even more useful in this regard if accompanied by a high intake of potassium-rich fruits and vegetables that buffers the acidifying impact of the protein."

We might add that some of the research currently underway on acidic diets, and their relationship to poor liver function, points to possible metabolic disturbances that are the result of such diets. The cortisol-endocrine link adds compelling evidence that our overly acidic diet needs to be neutralised not just by dietary changes but also by supplementation with alkaline minerals.

[15]

Why Supplementation with Alkaline Minerals Makes Sense

Given our Western lifestyle and the unlikelihood that most people will change their diet substantially, supplementation makes sense. However, we must distinguish between organic mineral supplements and inorganic mineral supplements, such as oxides and carbonates.

In the case of carbonates, the problem with ingesting something like sodium bicarbonate is that we reduce our stomach acid. This not only results in the production of carbon dioxide, with its potentially unpleasant effects, but it also increases the pH of the stomach. This is the one place in the body that we require an acidic pH, which is crucial for digestion. Without gastric acid, carbonates can't be used. In fact, one of the most common age-related causes of impaired digestive function is the reduction of hydrochloric acid produced by the stomach. Achlorhydria (the complete absence of stomach acid) and hypochlorhydria (low stomach acid) are common digestive problems (Kelly, 1997). Numerous studies have shown that hydrochloric acid secretion declines with advancing age. In one study, US researchers found that over 30% of men and women past the age of 60 suffer from atrophic gastritis, a condition marked by little or no acid secretion. A second study found that up to 40% of postmenopausal women have no basal gastric acid secretions. In another study involving 3,484 subjects, researchers found that among both males and females, 27% suffered from achlorhydria, with the greatest incidence (39.8%) occurring in females aged 80 to 89 years.

One of the important functions of HCl is that it aids in the absorption and assimilation of vitamins and minerals, such as folic acid, ascorbic acid, beta-carotene, and iron, by increasing their bioavailability and affecting their release from food. It has been shown that a number of minerals and trace elements are poorly absorbed in cases of low stomach acid, including calcium, magnesium, zinc, copper, chromium, selenium, manganese, vanadium, molybdenum, and cobalt. A reduction of an already low amount of gastric acid by neutralisation with carbonate supplements doesn't therefore make much sense.

When increased stomach acid is called for, this acid must be produced by the mucosa cells. Within these cells a reaction between water and carbon dioxide results in the production of acid and bicarbonate. The acid is secreted into the stomach, whereas the bicarbonate is secreted into the blood. The stomach acid then migrates to the intestines, where it's neutralised by the pancreatic fluid. Overall, this has no effect on the acid-base balance, since the acid produced in the stomach is neutralised by bicarbonate produced by the pancreas.

What this means in practice is that whenever we eat something, we saturate our periphery with blood that has a slightly higher bicarbonate content (in other words, an increased buffering capacity). Many people also take medications known as proton pump inhibitors to block the production of acid, which is far from a beneficial process and merely masks the problem of indigestion instead of addressing its cause. In this case, bicarbonate won't be dissolved. Over the long term, the addition of proton pump inhibitor medication adversely influences the functioning of the connective tissues, since it reduces the capacity of the body to remove the surplus of acid from these tissues. Even if HCl production is normal, the acid production in the stomach after taking a bicarbonate supplement will rapidly be replenished. In this case, there will be a fast increase of bicarbonate concentration in the blood, only to be excreted through the kidneys, giving us bicarbonate-rich urine. (By the way, this is the reason we have more-alkaline urine after taking these kinds of supplements). However, we don't want the beneficial alkalinity to be lost in the urine. We need it throughout the whole body so it has a chance to eliminate the surplus acid in the connective tissues. For these reasons, the addition of bicarbonate isn't the best way to alkaline supplement.

A much preferred approach utilises organic alkaline minerals, which consist principally of citrates. For example, potassium citrate dissociates into citric acid anion and potassium. The citric acid anion is the real alkalinising substance, since it carries a negative charge that can be used to bind protons—that is, to bind acid. This citric acid anion plus hydrogen (H+) becomes citric acid, which is metabolised mainly in the liver into water and carbon dioxide. One mole of citrate can bind three moles of acid. The kidneys must eliminate the magnesium, potassium, or sodium, which they do without problems, but they have difficulty with acid—something that's avoided when the acid is bound as to citrate, building citric acid.

The best alkaline supplementation is in the form of citrates: the sodium, potassium, calcium, and magnesium citrates. These salts neutralise gastric acid by only a minimal amount. We can take them without a negative effect on digestion. This is also convenient, since they don't have to be taken with a meal but can be ingested anytime. Also, potassium, calcium, and magnesium citrates are generally superior to sodium salts, as was found in the report cited earlier by Maurer et al. They conclude unequivocally that "studies that administered $NaHCO_3$ [sodium bicarbonate] and sodium citrate have found little effect on urinary calcium excretion...whereas those in which $KHCO_3$ or potassium citrate were administered have found large, significant reductions."

It takes a while for the alkalising effect of citrates to become overt, but the result is a steadier overall alkalisation, unlike the rapid rise and decrease caused by a bicarbonate supplement. To highlight the key concerns, bicarbonate leads to carbon dioxide formation in the stomach, which neutralises gastric acid and changes the stomach pH. This is a particular concern for the elderly, who in many cases already suffer from reduced acid production capacity and the resultant problem of the inhibition of the release of micronutrients from their food. Plus, the taste of bicarbonate isn't very pleasant. With citrate, there's good absorption of minerals, a long-lasting effect, and it's tasteless (which helps with compliance, since people won't take something over a long period if the taste is unpleasant).

We evolved on an alkaline diet, but now eat a highly acidic diet. We suggest that we at least need to return to a neutral diet if we are to achieve a positive long-term effect on our wellbeing

Dear reader, we hope to have convinced you that an adequate acid-base balance is of utmost importance for our general health and wellbeing. Sufficient intake of organic anions, like citrates, also automatically increases the intake of minerals. Chemically, it's impossible to ingest for instance citrates as anions alone. We always ingest citrate as a salt, mainly as potassium, sodium, calcium, or magnesium citrate. So, with alkaline supplementation there are two sides to the coin—intake of anions and intake of minerals. Increased alkalinity therefore also means increased intake of minerals. The second part of this book will show you that there is one mineral you should especially focus upon—magnesium. The importance of magnesium for our bodies is so crucial that it's surprising how neglected this amazing mineral was during the last century of research. Some scientists even refer to magnesium as the "forgotten ion." During recent years, however, many new aspects of magnesium have been discovered, and it was found that this essential mineral, in particular, has a tremendous impact on our disease risks, as well as our life expectancy.

[16]

Magnesium – Life's Essential Mineral

Magnesium is found widely in nature. Indeed, it's the eighth most common element in the earth's crust. So it's not surprising we also find a high concentration of this element in the oceans—55 mmol per litre. (In the Dead Sea in Israel, the concentration of magnesium is extremely high, nearly 200 mmol per litre.) Since life evolved in seawater, quite simply, magnesium has been present throughout our evolution, with the result that no cell on earth can live without it. In virtually no physiological process is this mineral unneeded (Vormann, 2012).

The human body contains around 25 grams of magnesium, distributed in such a way that a little more than half is found in our bones—53% to be precise. The bones act as a storage facility for magnesium.

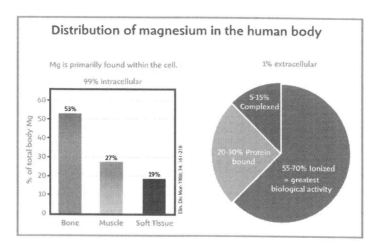

Figure 29: Distribution of magnesium

[17]

The Main Physiological Functions of Magnesium

One of the most important functions of magnesium is in it's join with ATP (adenosine triphosphate), which is our intracellular fuel. This fuel is active in the form of the ATP-magnesium complex. If we take magnesium away, we can't use our ATP, which means that an intracellular magnesium deficiency leads to an energy deficit in the cells. Magnesium is also crucial to the mitochondria, which are a membrane-enclosed structures found in cells. The mitochondria function as "cellular power plants," generating ATP.

Although allowing us to use intracellular fuel is a fundamental function of magnesium, it's far from the only function of this vital mineral. For instance, magnesium is also a physiological antagonist to calcium and functions as a cofactor in more than 300 enzymes. As such, it's essential to various structural proteins, as well as the structure of nucleic acids. Many important enzymes require the proper concentration of intracellular free magnesium, and the body utilises a variety of regulatory protocols to maintain the optimum concentration in our cells. But magnesium's extracellular function is also important.

In recent years magnesium has emerged as extremely important for the functioning of insulin, which means there's a close connection between magnesium and diabetes.

Further, it's known that magnesium has anti-apoptotic properties, which influence the processes involved in cancer. Probably because of its function in cell adhesion, magnesium deficiency plays an evident role in the spread of the cancer cells.

[18]

How Magnesium Works

How does magnesium work? There are several different mechanisms.

A cell membrane has a great many negative charges. As a divalent cation (an atom missing two electrons compared with a neutral atom), magnesium has two positive charges. By acting as a ligand—that is, a means of binding to two negative charges—magnesium stabilises the cell membrane, by cross-linking these charges.

If we eliminate magnesium or have a low extracellular concentration—in other words, a low concentration of magnesium in the blood—these charges will bind to sodium or potassium instead of magnesium. Both sodium and potassium are monovalent ions that cannot cross-link the membrane. Thus, if we take magnesium out of the picture, we destabilise the cell membrane. This has especially important repercussions for the nervous system.

In a cell, magnesium is able to enter a calcium channel—although it's too big to pass through the channel. The result is that a certain percentage of the body's calcium channels are blocked by magnesium. The block isn't permanent but, as we shall see, serves a purpose for a time. The availability of calcium channels is determined by the quantity of magnesium present in the plasma.

This is a particularly important function of magnesium, given that calcium is used as a second messenger. Calcium channels are intimately linked with sodium channels in the cell membrane, which send a signal to the cell to release the stress hormones, adrenaline and noradrenaline. The rapidity of this response, and the payload delivered, is greatly influenced by the amount of magnesium present. If a person has a magnesium deficiency, the calcium channel will transfer its signal more rapidly, thus releasing an excess of stress hormones—and doing so far more rapidly than were magnesium sufficiently present in the channel to partially block it and thereby regulate the rate of release. In other words, a high magnesium concentration slows the process, which means that magnesium is a natural anti-stress mineral—a truly important function and of particular significance for individuals in a stressed state.

A sufficient magnesium intake is crucial for the regulation of its homeostasis. Daily dietary intake of magnesium should be at least 300 milligrams, preferably more toward 420 milligrams, with 360 as a mean. Generally, only about a third of the magnesium we take in is absorbed in our intestines, with two-thirds remaining in the intestines—which is why an excess of some forms of magnesium in particular can cause diarrhoea. After absorption, the blood distributes magnesium to the other cells; and if there is an increase, then the other cells can also fulfil their magnesium needs.

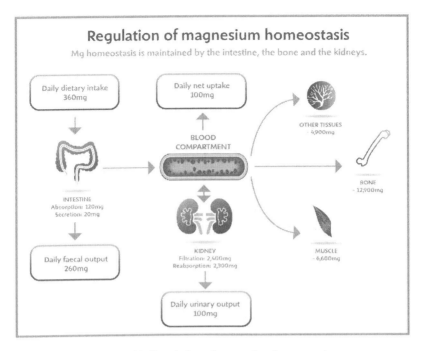

Figure 30: Regulation of magnesium homeostasis

The kidneys are the main organs in terms of regulating the homeostasis of magnesium in our bodies. Some 2,400 milligrams of magnesium are ultra-filtrated out of the blood by the kidneys on a daily basis, 95% of which must be reabsorbed from the primary urine. An adequate dietary intake provides us with a net uptake of around 100 milligrams from the intestines, one third of the daily dietary intake. To be in a steady state, or what we refer to as "homeostasis," we must excrete just these 100 milligrams, which we do through the urine. This means the individual has to reabsorb 2,300 milligrams of the 2,400 milligrams that enter the kidneys with the ultra-filtrate from blood. Hence, the kidneys fulfil a vital role in regulating the amount of magnesium in the body. Everything that influences kidney function also influences the homeostasis of magnesium.

[19]

How Magnesium is Absorbed by the Body

During recent years, the mechanisms by which magnesium is absorbed in the intestines and reabsorbed in the kidneys have become clear (De Baaij et al, 2015). Having said this, we need to point out that when it comes to science, it's always more complicated than the simple statement that something is "clear." With this proviso in mind, several mechanisms are nevertheless known to us.

We have two different pathways for the absorption of magnesium. The first is via para-cellular pathways, which are a pathway that crosses a layer **between** cells, and for this we need the so-called claudins—proteins that decide whether magnesium can pass into the blood. These proteins are under the control of vitamin D. Thus, a vitamin D deficiency affects the homeostasis of magnesium. Even if you receive a lot of sun, a deficiency of vitamin D isn't at all uncommon. Another pathway is trans-cellular, meaning transport **through** the cells. There are several cellular channels for magnesium uptake. Although these are the most important channels, other transporters also bring magnesium into the cell. However, we don't require magnesium only in the cells, we need it in the blood, and beyond.

For this, we need a different system. This is the so-called sodium-magnesium-antiport. Magnesium leaves the cell in exchange for sodium. It took us 25 years to learn the exact mechanism by which this operates. Only recently, in 2012, could we at last claim we have identified the gene that decides the amount of, what we refer to as, a "magnesium exchanger" in the cells (Kolisek et al., 2012). This is important because this sodium-magnesium exchanger is present in all cells in our body. It's the main magnesium efflux system. It's important to know that this system can become blocked by certain pharmacological substances, which inhibit the magnesium influx from the cell. One of the important functions of certain drugs is to keep magnesium in the cell. It was also found that this transporter might be genetically different in a subgroup of patients with Parkinson's disease, or might be differently regulated in conditions such as preeclampsia, as we have been able to show recently. Only now, knowing the genetic backgrounds of magnesium regulation, can there be more specific investigations into the contribution of this system to various diseases.

Magnesium must be reabsorbed in the glomerulus and the kidneys. Most is absorbed in the thick ascending limb (TAL), but also in the distal convoluted tubule (DCT), with something like 90-95% being retrieved in one of these two ways. The mechanism for this retrieval is similar to the mechanism that enables magnesium reabsorption in the intestines. Again, we have a para-cellular pathway and we have trans-cellular pathways, which involve several different genes that regulate the influx of magnesium into the cell.

A number of diseases are caused by inherited genetic defects. The human body has several magnesium transporters that regulate our magnesium status and hereditary defects in these magnesium transporters are known to cause some of these diseases.

On top of this, there is the question of whether people actually receive the ideal daily intake of something in the range of 300 to 420 milligrams of magnesium. Do most of us eat sufficient magnesium-rich foods? Nuts and seeds are rich in magnesium. So too are green vegetables and salads, which of course contain chlorophyll. In fact, everything that's green is full of magnesium because the green colour comes from chlorophyll, in which magnesium is the central ion. If we remove magnesium from chlorophyll, it loses its colour. While it's easy to diagnose a magnesium deficiency in plants precisely because they have a bleached appearance, it's not so easy in the case of humans. What a pity nature didn't make us green, like we once imagined inhabitants of Mars to be! Our work would have been so much easier.

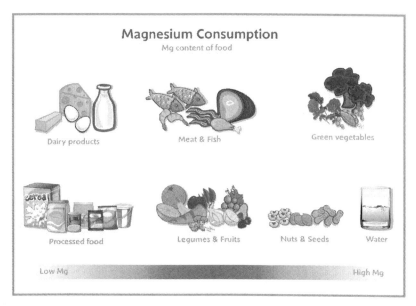

Figure 31: Magnesium consumption

Not only do we experience a low intake of magnesium from the food we choose to eat, but we also lose a lot in food preparation. Processed foods are notoriously low in magnesium, since all processing of food diminishes the magnesium content. For instance, simply boiling a potato extracts 50% of the magnesium, which is lost in the cooking water. And what do we do with the water? We usually throw it away. Today, of course, more and more of us are eating processed foods that contain little nutrition, and certainly little magnesium, so that magnesium deficiency is increasing.

In Australia, 41% of males and 35% of females in the age of 19 years and over obtain less than the recommended daily intake of magnesium. Low intakes were found especially in the age groups of 14-18 years, with 61% of males and 71 % of females not reaching the requirements. Also, aged people over 71 have low intake with a prevalence of inadequacy for men of 63% and women 48%. (Australian Health Survey, 2015)

Another study, this time conducted in 2008 in Germany, revealed that 26% of men and 28% of women have an intake of magnesium that's below the daily suggested requirement (Nationale Verzehrsstudie 2008).

If we examine the data for the different age groups, we discover that the incidence of low intake in females in their teens runs at 56%, double that of the average woman. One reason for this is that these are the years when young woman tend to indulge in dieting in an attempt to match up to Western society's stereotype of the ideal female body. It's also during the teen and young adult years that women tend to embark on pregnancy, with many of them starving themselves during the pregnancy to keep their figure, thereby greatly reducing their magnesium intake—a practice that's good for neither the mother nor the child.

Another German study from 1995 looked at the serum magnesium concentration (Kohlmeier et al., 1995). The threshold chosen in this study was extremely conservative, deeming females to be deficient in magnesium only if their level was below 0.67 mM. Today, a minimum level to maintain one's health is considered to be 0.75 mM, with 0.85 mM and above the optimum. By today's standards, the incidence of magnesium deficiency would be much higher. But even using the conservative levels of the 1995 study, a low plasma magnesium concentration was evident in about 10% of the population but the incidence was double in women age 18 to 24.

Additional problems occur as we age. We mentioned that our bones serve as our magnesium storehouse. A study, conducted by us, measured the magnesium concentration in the bones of traffic accident victims (Vormann and Anke, 2002). It demonstrated that the older people become, the lower the magnesium content of their bones. When we are elderly, we don't have a good store of magnesium. We also lose our ability to release magnesium from our bones efficiently. Because the process takes longer, it becomes more difficult to maintain a consistent serum magnesium level.

Crucial to this whole picture is the fact that our acid-base affects our magnesium balance. One of our studies, some years ago now, determined the urinary net acid excretion as a parameter of an individual's acid-base status (Rylander et al., 2006). We saw the higher the acid excretion, the higher the urinary magnesium loss.

It is now known simply by ageing we slide into a latent acidosis, due to reduced kidney function, which drives magnesium out of the body. This may be the reason the magnesium stores in our bones decrease as we age.

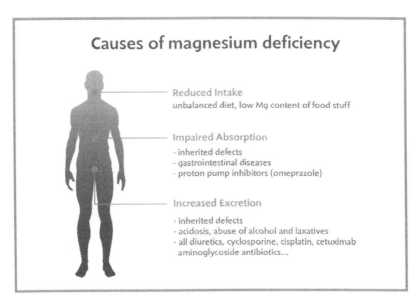

Figure 32: Causes of magnesium deficiency

Humans vary in their ability to absorb magnesium. Some have no difficulty with magnesium uptake, while others with a lower absorption capacity slip into a deficit much earlier in life. Part of this may be due to so-called polymorphisms of the genes involved in magnesium regulation. Tiny changes in efficacy of production of magnesium regulating systems might influence the ability of an individual to stay in balance. A variety of gastrointestinal diseases also play a part in reducing our ability to absorb magnesium. Generally, all diseases or infections leading to diarrhoea will tremendously reduce the ability to absorb magnesium from the intestines. An often-overlooked side effect of proton pump inhibitors is to lower our ability to release magnesium from our food. Long-term intake of these proton pump inhibitors has been known to induce severe magnesium deficiency. These proton pump inhibitors reduce the production of gastric acid, and if we don't produce sufficient gastric acid, magnesium simply isn't released from food or from some supplements. Magnesium that isn't bioavailable is then excreted. Indeed, one of the most important factors in the induction of magnesium deficiency is increased excretion via the faecal or urinary route.

Alcohol also increases magnesium excretion, since alcohol is a diuretic. Alcohol abuse is a major cause of magnesium deficiency. Whenever you seen an alcoholic with shaky hands, the shaking is mainly due to a lack of magnesium. The smart thing is to drink less, while also increasing your magnesium intake. (Should you wish to visit Munich during Oktoberfest, you'd be wise to take plenty of magnesium before you imbibe. You'll certainly fare better the next day, since magnesium is an antidote to hangovers! But you do have to take it in advance to get the maximum benefit, as we can testify from experience).

Many widely used drugs influence kidney function. Diuretics, whether they are potassium sparing or not, influence magnesium status (Lameris et al., 2012). Increased diuresis drives magnesium out of the body. Cyclosporine, a substance all transplant patients must take the rest of their lives, is an extremely strong inhibitor of the magnesium reuptake systems in the kidneys, which is particularly poignant since all transplant patients need high doses of magnesium (though unfortunately they don't get the right amount, as most doctors are unaware of this). The same is true of cancer therapies, such as Cisplatin and Cetuximab, both of which are used especially in colon cancer therapy but induce dramatic magnesium deficits by inhibiting reabsorption in the kidneys. Antibiotics, in particular aminoglycoside antibiotics, also inhibit reuptake of magnesium in the kidneys. Consequently, all patients taking these antibiotics require magnesium supplementation.

We have covered the problem of gastrointestinal malabsorption, but there are also endocrine causes of hypomagnesemia. (When we speak of too low a plasma-magnesium concentration, keep in mind that plasma and serum is the same thing when it comes to magnesium).

Another cause of magnesium deficiency is stress. Stress will induce cellular magnesium losses, leading to a short-lived increase in plasma magnesium concentration. This increase will be normalised by increased urinary excretion, however, the reuptake of intracellular magnesium will reduce plasma magnesium and at the end, a magnesium deficit remains. Long-lasting stressful periods are therefore a major cause of magnesium deficiency, as long as reasonable magnesium supplementation doesn't keep up with the losses (Seelig 1994).

Excessive sweating can also lead to significant loss, which is why athletes are smart to take magnesium. However, the content of magnesium in sweat decreases if we sweat a lot. For instance, soccer players lose more magnesium when they start training than when they are in a trained phase. Nevertheless, it's important to realise that we lose significant amounts of magnesium when we sweat, and take steps to replace it. But note that magnesium supplements should be taken in the regeneration phase and not directly before a competition. Too much magnesium could slow down the reaction phase somewhat (which you don´t want when running a 100 metre sprint) or induce some softening of stool (which is also not very pleasant when running a marathon, for example).

[20]

How to Recognise
Magnesium Deficiency

What are the main symptoms of magnesium deficiency? Unfortunately, there's no single obvious symptom. It's not as simple as saying, "I have a cramp." If you have a cramp, it's likely you do have a deficiency, but that's far from the most important symptom of a deficiency.

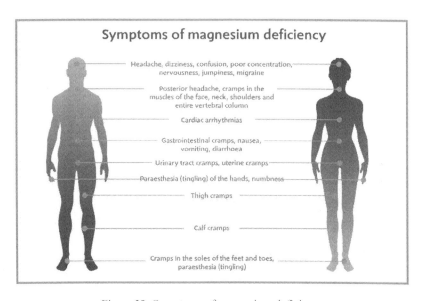

Figure 33: Symptoms of magnesium deficiency

Magnesium deficiency can result in headaches, dizziness, nervousness, confusion, poor concentration, migraines, and cramp in the muscles of the face, neck, shoulders, and the entire vertebral column. Indeed, cramps anywhere in the body can be connected to a deficiency of magnesium. But adequate magnesium isn't only a means of avoiding such things as calf cramps. Rather, it's truly essential for life. The fact is, because a magnesium deficiency is related to many diseases, it manifests in quite a variety of symptoms.

Having said there are no obvious indicators, we should add that a high percentage of cardiac arrhythmias are due to magnesium deficiency. Another small but strong indicator of a deficiency is tingling of the eyelid. If you find your eyelid tingling, you can assume your magnesium is low, and doctors are wise to watch for this in patients.

The majority of medical patients are hypomagnesaemic (have low serum magnesium concentration)—although the condition isn't generally identified because doctors don't tend to test for this. It's not currently part of the clinical routine (Whang and Ryder, 1990). Despite the lack of testing, studies show that only a minority of patients whose magnesium status is tested fall within the optimal range of concentration, which is 0.85 to 1.1 mmol per litre. Only a tiny number have higher values. Again, the clinical signs of hypomagnesaemia are nonspecific and can show up either in the neuromuscular area, the central nervous system, the metabolic system, or especially the cardiovascular system.

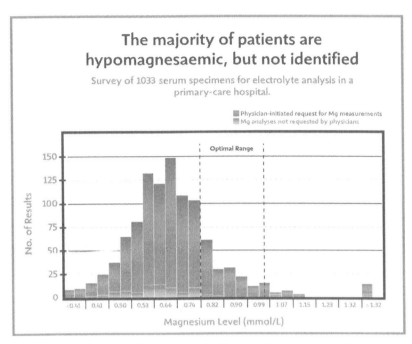

Figure 34: The majority of patients are hypomagnesaemic

We have very convincing data on the importance of magnesium for the cardiovascular system. In a small yet poignant study, fourteen women received a diet with only 100 milligrams of magnesium for up to 78 days to induce magnesium deficiency (Nielsen et al., 2007). Since this is generally unethical, it wasn't easy to get the study approved by the ethical committees. The FDA in the United States ultimately sanctioned it, since the point was that if 25% of the American population eats only about 100 milligrams of magnesium on a daily basis, we should be able to duplicate the effects in a clinical setting and see what the effects may be.

The fourteen women selected for the study were closely monitored. In five of them, severe cardiac arrhythmias occurred. Of course, when the arrhythmias were detected, magnesium supplementation was administered, and the arrhythmias disappeared. None of the women experienced a cramp in their calf, yet a third of them experienced cardiac arrhythmias, which confirms that arrhythmia is a good indicator of a magnesium deficiency.

[21]

Your Heart and Brain are at Risk

We can treat cardiac arrhythmias with magnesium supplementation. In fact, studies show oral magnesium supplementation has the same effect as a magnesium infusion through the blood, in terms of resumption of a normal cardiac rhythm in patients undergoing cardiac surgery. Surprisingly, oral supplementation has even shown itself to be somewhat superior. Since the reduction of arrhythmias can be accomplished, at least as effectively with oral doses of magnesium as with intravenous infusion, this simplifies treatment.

Similarly, we have seen in studies of both men and women that there's a significant correlation between decreased plasma magnesium concentration and the risk of sudden cardiac death (Chiuve et al., 2011). Quite simply, we can avoid up to three quarters of sudden cardiac deaths by ensuring an individual has the correct concentration of magnesium. In other words, in some cases your magnesium status literally determines whether you live or die of sudden cardiac failure.

In a recent study from Germany, 4,230 individuals were followed over a period of twelve years (Reffelmann et al., 2011). The subjects were divided into two groups according to their plasma magnesium concentration, with the split determined by those above 0.73 mmol per litre and those below. The group with the low magnesium concentration experienced a mortality rate significantly higher than the group with the higher concentration. Again, the evidence shows that magnesium is a determining factor in how long you live.

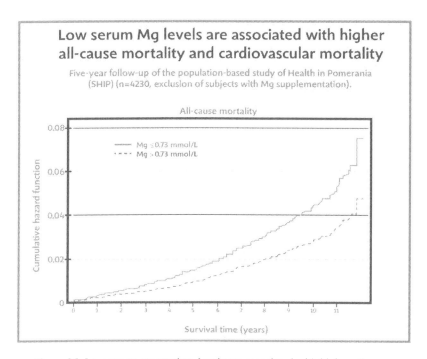

Figure 35: Low serum magnesium levels are associated with higher all-cause mortality and cardiovascular mortality

Magnesium status is also inversely associated with the risk of stroke. Studies have shown that you can reduce your risk of stroke by about 50% by having an appropriate concentration of magnesium in your body (Larsson et al., 2012). Indeed, in a meta-analysis of prospective studies it was found that an increase of 100 milligrams of magnesium per day results in a 10% decrease in the risk of stroke.

The fact is, magnesium also greatly reduces the occurrence of atherosclerosis. The higher the concentration of magnesium in the body, the lower the risk of any form of coronary heart disease. As a recently published meta-analysis revealed (Qu et al., 2013), in the vast majority of studies that were considered, increased serum magnesium concentrations resulted in a reduction in risk of total cardiovascular events. Only a small number of studies failed to reflect this, in contrast to the overwhelming majority of studies. This is extremely important, given that the majority of us fall into the sector of the population in which serum magnesium concentrations are relatively low. In particular, women can avoid nearly two-thirds of all cardiovascular disease—the percentage isn't quite as high in males. Women especially profit from a high plasma magnesium concentration.

Another recent and rather large study of the correlation of dietary magnesium and plasma magnesium concentration and the risk of coronary heart disease followed 86,000 women for up to 28 years (Chiuve et al., 2013). The data shows that there is only a small risk reduction with increased magnesium intake if you look at the incidence of total cardiovascular events. However, if you differentiate into non-fatal and fatal coronary heart disease, there is a stunning result. Non-fatal heart disease is nearly uninfluenced by increased magnesium intake, whereas there is a clear and significant negative correlation of increased magnesium intake with fatal heart disease in this population of women. This result simply shows that it is your magnesium status that decides whether you survive a cardiac attack. So it's a wise idea to avoid a magnesium deficit whenever you can—something that isn't too complicated, as we will see later.

There are now many studies of large numbers of people that show the change of relative risk of cardiovascular disease if you have, for instance, 0.2 mmol per litre higher plasma magnesium. You can reduce your cardiovascular disease risk by 30% simply by increasing your level of circulating magnesium. In the case of ischemic heart disease, there is a risk reduction of 17% when magnesium circulating in the blood is high, with a whopping 40% less cases of fatality in the case of ischemic heart attacks.

In other words, the higher your magnesium intake, the lower your risk of acquiring coronary heart disease, and the greater your chances of surviving a heart attack if you are unfortunately enough to experience one. This is just further evidence that, as a general health practice, we should aim to ensure a high plasma magnesium concentration in the entire population—the higher, the better.

In the case of coronary heart disease, using magnesium to treat patients can greatly reduce the need for other treatments such as calcium channel blockers, beta blockers, and nitrates (Wilimzig and Vierling, 1991). Indeed, we find supplementing a patient's magnesium to be extremely effective when it comes to their overall functionality.

[22]

Magnesium and Diabetes

Many diabetics have reduced magnesium content in their serum. In fact, the incidence of hypomagnesaemia in type 2 diabetics is much higher than in their healthy counterparts. The reason is that diabetics have polyuria and simply lose a lot of magnesium in their urine daily.

Magnesium status is also closely related to a risk of becoming diabetic in the first place. The higher the daily magnesium intake, the lower the risk of developing diabetes. For instance, in a meta-analysis of seven prospective cohort studies, with over 600,000 subjects involved, about a 15% reduction of risk with each 100-milligram increase in daily intake of magnesium was found (Larsson and Wolk, 2007).

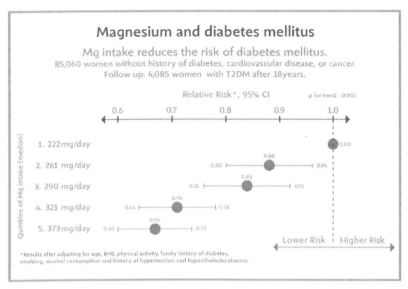

Figure 36: Magnesium and diabetes mellitus

So, magnesium is extremely protective against developing type two diabetes. This was also shown in a study by a friend of ours in Mexico, Professor Fernando Guerrero-Romero, who along with others conducted a 10-year follow-up study on plasma magnesium concentration in the population and correlated it with the percentage of the population who developed diabetes mellitus (Guerrero-Romero and Rodríguez-Morán, 2006). The lower the plasma concentration, the higher the risk of becoming diabetic up to a factor of five. What we also see from this study is that if you have a high plasma magnesium concentration, you can just about completely avoid the risk of developing diabetes.

Another large epidemiological study, the already mentioned Nurses Health Study, demonstrated that a large increase of magnesium resulted in a significant reduction in the risk of diabetes, up to some 40%.

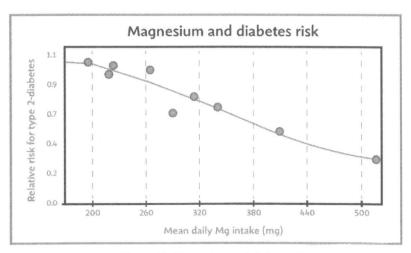

Figure 37: Magnesium and diabetes risk

A study from Australia (Simmons et al., 2010) contrasts those who don't take antihypertensive medication with those who do. Patients on antihypertensives have seven times more often hypomagnesemia than controls. In comparison to these normal healthy adults, patients newly diagnosed as diabetic have an even higher incidence of hypomagnesaemia, which increases by a factor of ten.

A meta-analysis of studies involving several hundred thousand people also show that the relative risk of developing diabetes is significantly reduced by increased magnesium intake (Kim et al., 2010). For instance, with only a 100 milligram daily increase, the risk goes down by 15%. This is a very small increase in magnesium intake, and greater quantities decrease the risk considerably more effectively. In our professional opinion, we would say that by doubling your intake of magnesium you can reduce your relative risk by 50%.

What's the chemistry behind this? During recent years, much has been learned on this subject.

Magnesium significantly influences the insulin status and the function of insulin in our bodies. In patients with hypomagnesemia, we find diminished glucose transport capacity as the sensitivity of the insulin receptor is established by sufficient magnesium. But also insulin secretion is below normal. Additionally, we find impairment in the post-receptor insulin signalling cascade. In sum, what happens intracellularly when insulin works on a cell is intensively influenced by the individual's magnesium status.

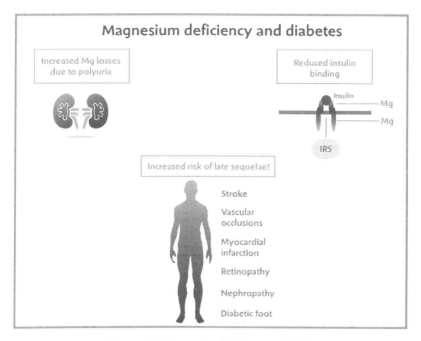

Figure 38: Magnesium deficiency and diabetes

A study of oral magnesium supplementation in elderly diabetic patients, especially focusing on their vascular function, resulted in a dramatic increase in flow-mediated dilation in the magnesium supplemented group (Barbagallo et al., 2010). This is a good parameter for the overall functioning of the vasculature. In the control group, there was no change from the baseline after a month. This leads us to conclude that high-dose magnesium supplementation has a positive effect on vascular health in diabetics. This makes sense, given that the problems with diabetics relate mainly to blood flow through the organs and the late complications that result in these patients. We have clear evidence that the system can be significantly improved with proper magnesium supplementation.

Also, pre-diabetic patients—those with metabolic syndrome—benefitted from daily magnesium supplementation. A randomised, double-blind, placebo-controlled study (Guerrero-Romera et a., 2004) done in Mexico, showed that when pre-diabetics receive high doses of magnesium, glucose goes down—especially haemoglobin A1C, which is a clinically relevant effect. The capacity to produce insulin is also improved, and the HOMA-IR index goes down—a considerably improved situation.

We need to mention that patients received 2.5 grams of magnesium chloride per day. You might wonder why magnesium chloride was used. Well, it was the only type of magnesium available in Mexico at that time. Although it's not the ideal, it nevertheless worked. The dose was high, delivering 600 milligrams of magnesium. The problem is that it tastes horrible! Once you taste magnesium chloride, you're unlikely to take it for long.

We are currently doing a number of studies with the same Mexican researchers, at The Institute of Diabetes Research. In the newer studies, we have exchanged magnesium chloride for magnesium citrate. Magnesium citrate tastes better, which increases compliance. There's another factor that comes into play with magnesium chloride: it induces a state of acidosis in the body. Whenever a person takes either magnesium chloride or calcium chloride, they induce acidosis. Hence neither of these are the optimal delivery method for magnesium supplementation. In contrast, magnesium citrate is an alkalising substance, which benefits the body in a variety of ways. This is extremely important particularly for diabetics, as they often develop acute acidosis. With proper magnesium supplementation, a person can avoid hypomagnesaemia as well as acidosis.

When looking at meta-analyses, we have to be cautious in drawing definite conclusions, since there are studies that show a positive effect and others that don't. However, when we examine the studies in detail, we find those that showed a negative effect were studies in which they used magnesium preparations that aren't well absorbed. The dosage was also extremely low. A failure to compare apples with apples and oranges with oranges is frequently a problem with studies. It's crucial to compare things that offer a legitimate comparison, both in the type of substance used and the dosage. In the case of those studies that show supplementation to be extremely effective, all used high doses of the optimum form of magnesium. So it's extremely important which kind of magnesium salt is used, and of course in what dosage.

We need to mention one other study from the same group in Mexico, because it addresses what we believe to be a common problem—diabetics who also suffer from depression. In this study, one group took magnesium, while the other group took the antidepressant Imipramine (Barragán-Rodríguez et al., 2008). The antidepressant clearly worked, with the depression score falling from 16 to around 11 on the scale. However, and this is something that was quite surprising, magnesium supplementation proved to be just as effective.

A factor we must consider is that we were able to show a long time ago that Imipramine inhibits the efflux of magnesium from the cells. If this happens in neural cells, the intracellular magnesium levels stay high. So even in the case of the antidepressant, magnesium is involved. But the great news is that a sufficiently high dose of magnesium can achieve the same effect without any of the side effects with which long-term intake of this antidepressant drug is often connected.

The main point of this study is that magnesium obviously has a fundamental effect on the nervous system. One of its most important functions is to physiologically block the NMDA receptor, which has a magnesium binding site that's in equilibrium with magnesium outside the cells. The higher our magnesium intake, and the higher our plasma magnesium concentration, the more the receptor is blocked.

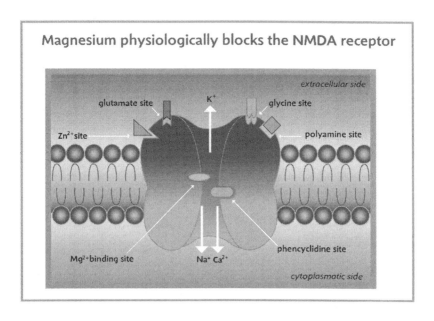

Figure 39: Magnesium physiologically blocks the NMDA receptor

Of course, we don't want the receptor to be completely blocked, since an over-excitation of this receptor isn't beneficial to us. For example, we require low activity in these receptors for learning and memory. Though we so far don't have human studies on this, a study from animal experiments is illuminating (Hoane 2011). These animals received either a normal diet of magnesium or a magnesium-deficient diet. The learning and memory capability was much lower in the magnesium-deficient group.

[23]

Magnesium and Neurological Issues

A recent discovery concerns magnesium and Alzheimer's disease. In patients with Alzheimer's, the ionized magnesium levels in plasma are reduced (Barbagallo et al., 2011). We also know that the trafficking and processing of the amyloid-beta protein responsible for the problems associated with Alzheimer's is significantly influenced by magnesium (Yu et al., 2010). When there is a magnesium deficiency, this protein precipitates much earlier than with higher concentrations of magnesium. Also, low serum magnesium levels correlate with clinical deterioration in Alzheimer's disease (Cilliler et al., 2007). By avoiding low magnesium intake (and acidosis, of course), we give ourselves some protection against this devastating disease.

Another important area in which magnesium plays an important role is Parkinson's disease. In Germany alone, some 300,000 people suffer from Parkinson's today. This represents a dramatic increase in recent years. But how might magnesium help? It's known that magnesium in vitro has both preventive and ameliorating effects in rats (Hashimoto et al., 2008). It's also known that certain genes contains genetic variants in Parkinson's disease patients (Yan et al., 2011). One of these genes is the SLC41A1 gene, which as we can show encodes for the sodium-magnesium exchanger. This system takes magnesium out of the cell. The problem with Parkinson's patients might be that they have a magnesium efflux that's more active than we find in individuals who don't have this genetic defect.

We can speculate that Parkinson's is connected to a change in the intracellular magnesium homeostasis.

Another neurological issue is the problem of headaches, especially migraines. We have known for some time that the magnesium concentration in the plasma, blood cells, saliva, cerebrospinal fluid, and cerebral cortex is reduced in those who experience migraines. In one study, the intracellular ionized magnesium in the brain was measured using nuclear magnetic resonance, which is a fairly complex process and not something that can be done routinely (Lodi et al., 2001). The concentration of magnesium was high in the control group, but low in the group suffering from migraines. Concerning different severities of migraines it was shown that the greater the severity of the migraine, the lower the free magnesium concentration in the brain.

A study using 600 milligrams of magnesium as Magnesium-Diasporal®, a brand name pharmaceutical grade magnesium citrate often used in our studies, over a period of twelve weeks, showed a significant reduction in the frequency of migraine attacks (Peikert et al., 1996).

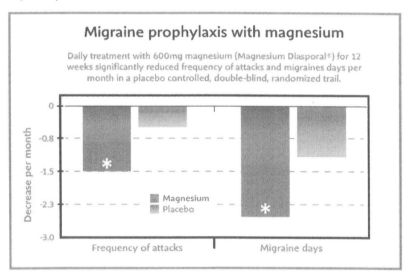

Figure 40: Migraine prophylaxis with magnesium

This study was later repeated, again using supplementation of 600 milligrams per day over twelve weeks (Köseoglu et al., 2008). In the placebo group, there was no change in the intensity of pain. In contrast, in the group supplemented with magnesium the pain intensity was considerably reduced—in fact, almost halved.

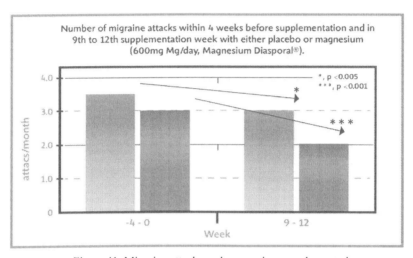

Figure 41: Migraine attacks and magnesium supplementation

We wish to emphasise that this was the effect for a group of patients. However, we now know that we have responders and non-responders. It's generally the case that around 50% of migraine patients respond to magnesium supplementation extremely well, whereas others don't respond. We also want to emphasise that you need a high dose. Some subjects who experienced 600 milligrams with no effect were given higher doses. If 900 milligrams had no effect, we tried 1200 milligrams, which produced some effect. However, at 1500 milligrams the migraines were gone. It's a question of titrating the patient according to their specific need.

At these larger doses, we have to consider possible side effects. The only side effect that can occur is the loosening of stool to the point of causing diarrhoea. It's therefore unwise to begin supplementation with too large a dose at once. For instance, we might start with 400 milligrams. Of course, for some with constipation, the loosening effect of magnesium is a welcome side effect. But about 10-15% of individuals will experience too much loosening at even 400 milligrams.

Thankfully, people tend to become accustomed to magnesium supplementation, which allows us to increase the dose. A person might begin on 400 milligrams, have no adverse reaction, and increase from there—in the case of someone whose migraines continue, perhaps going to 800 milligrams next, split over two doses at different times of day. If the person tolerates this amount, the dosage can be increased further if necessary.

When people can't tolerate more than 400 milligrams, there are two possible approaches. One is to add the second dosage only on alternate days, so that one day they receive 400 milligrams and the next 800 milligrams in two doses. The second is to dissolve the magnesium citrate in water and consume it over the course of the day, a sip at a time. Distributed throughout the waking day, the higher dosage becomes more tolerable. So if you find you have stomach or intestinal problems, sip your magnesium all day.

Patients with hereditary magnesium wasting need to take tremendously high amounts. Some require between 3,000 and 4,000 milligrams on a daily basis, which is the only way for them to remain in balance. Thankfully, genetically determined magnesium wasting is rare. The point is that patients' needs are all individual and need to be titrated accordingly.

A group at the New York Headache Center of Cornell University published a paper entitled "Why all migraine patients should be treated with magnesium" (Mauskop and Varughese, 2012). The paper suggests that deficiency is present in up to half of migraine sufferers and concludes that oral supplementation is warranted for all who experience migraines. In many cases this allows many patients to avoid taking medications that have severe side effects. Having mentioned side effects, we should add that the side effects of many drugs are significantly increased when magnesium concentrations are low. Many drugs reduce the capacity of the kidneys to reabsorb magnesium. A magnesium deficit is worsened in patients taking drugs, since many drugs work by increasing the calcium influx into the cells—an unwelcome side effect of such drugs. If magnesium concentrations are low, magnesium's ability to mitigate this situation is inhibited, which is how the side effects of the drugs can increase.

Magnesium is also effective in patients with tension headaches. In one study, 40 individuals from a special headache clinic, all of whom had suffered from tension headaches for years, consumed 600 milligrams of magnesium supplementation per day for two months (Taubert and Keil, 1991). The results were dramatic, with some of them even becoming free of headaches.

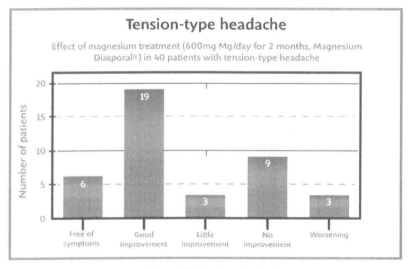

Figure 42: Tension headache

We need to emphasise that it can take two to three months to refill our magnesium stores, which of course are the bones. If the bone is tremendously depleted of magnesium, a significant increase in plasma magnesium concentration will only occur after some weeks of supplementation. Only then are we likely to see a reduction of headache attacks.

Magnesium is effective for asthma, too, relieving the bronchi. In a randomised crossover study with asthma patients, who were treated orally with 400 milligrams of magnesium per day for three weeks alongside a group who were given a placebo, the symptom index dropped significantly, with zero change in the placebo group (Hill et al., 1997). The use of a bronchial dilator also dropped significantly. Other studies done to the highest standards further confirm that magnesium makes a considerable difference (Kazaks et al., 2010).

[24]

Magnesium and Pregnancy

During the course of a pregnancy, there is a reduction of the concentration of plasma magnesium. In part, this is connected to the dilution of the plasma, but also the need of the child as it's fed from the mother.

Reduced magnesium concentration during pregnancy has negative effects, some of which are serious. For instance, there's an increase in the rate of spontaneous abortion, as well as preterm births. We also see a reduced birth weight and impaired development of the foetus. In the mother, there can be pregnancy-induced hypertension, pre-eclampsia, and other disorders. The mother often also experiences frequent leg cramps and symptoms such as headaches, double or blurred vision, and abdominal pressure and nausea.

In a clinical trial involving 568 women, the group who received magnesium supplementation experienced a reduced number of days in hospital, less haemorrhaging, a reduction of premature labour from 8.2% to 2.8%, a lower number of cases of cervical insufficiency, and a slightly increased duration of pregnancy (Spätling and Spätling, 1988). The incidence of women experiencing premature labour was greatly reduced simply by supplementing with magnesium. There were also positive effects for the child, including a reduction in premature births, less need for intensive neonatal care, normalising of birth weight, and increased body length. The total hospitalisation in the magnesium group was significantly lower than for the placebo group.

Eclampsia is perhaps the most serious problem of pregnancy, connected to significant morbidity and mortality for both mother and child. Although the treatment of choice worldwide for eclampsia is magnesium infusion, sadly pregnant women don't receive oral magnesium supplementation on a global scale—with one exception, which is Germany, where more than two-thirds of pregnant women take magnesium.

Because of the high level of magnesium supplementation in Germany, which would have skewed our results, we conducted a study in Sweden, a country in which magnesium supplementation is largely unheard of (Bullarbo et al., 2013). 60 women were part of the placebo-controlled study, all of them with an increased risk for pregnancy-induced hypertension. During the last three months of pregnancy, magnesium citrate was administered at a rate of 300 milligrams a day. Of 71 women who received no intervention, 18 experienced an increase of blood pressure. In the placebo group, 9 of the 29 candidates experienced increased hypertension. But in the group that received the magnesium, only 1 in 24 experienced an increase in blood pressure. We also measured the gene expression of various magnesium sensitive genes, which further revealed the effectiveness of this study.

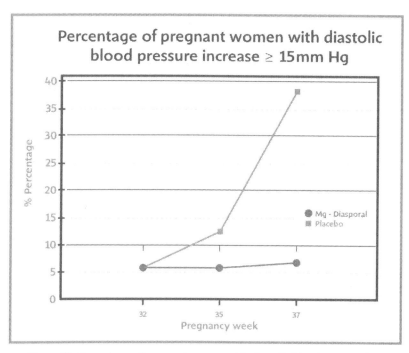

Figure 43: Percentage of pregnant women with diastolic blood pressure increase

Our intention now is to conduct a study of pregnant women in Sweden, Tanzania, Mexico, and China, which will allow us to investigate whether magnesium supplementation can significantly reduce pre-eclampsia, since this is such a serious issue. The incidence of pre-eclampsia in Sweden, where living conditions are extremely good, is very low at 3%. In Tanzania, the incidence runs around 25%. China has an incidence of about 15% and Mexico around 20%. If we could avoid this problem, as the data so far indicates we can, it would be of tremendous benefit. It should also not be forgotten that excessive lactation during certain phases of breast feeding can result in a considerable loss of magnesium.

[25]

Other Benefits of Magnesium for Women

Magnesium can be used in women with dysmenorrhoea (painful menstruation, especially abdominal cramps). In an observational study of 64 women, high oral magnesium supplementation, at a rate of 600 milligrams a day, significantly improved the clinical symptoms of this affliction (Wilimzig and Pannewig, 1994).

Another area in which magnesium has a positive effect is osteoporosis. Magnesium was used in a study to see if it could suppress bone turnover in postmenopausal osteoporotic women (Aydin et al., 2010). In the control group, osteocalcin (which is a marker of bone turnover) remained more or less unchanged, whereas magnesium supplementation produced a positive increase. Bone degradation was also reduced in the magnesium group compared with the control group.

Magnesium, especially magnesium citrate, is extremely important when it comes to osteoporosis. The citrate form not only assists us with absorbing magnesium, but also helps us avoid over-acidification, which is extremely detrimental to bone. By supplementing with magnesium citrate, we win on both counts.

[26]

When Magnesium is the Wrong Thing to Give

Are there situations in which magnesium is contraindicated, or even dangerous? For instance, should some individuals not be given magnesium supplementation?

There are people who have severe kidney dysfunction, and therefore should avoid magnesium supplements (Coburn et al., 1969). When a person is in stages four or five of chronic kidney disease, we find an increase in plasma magnesium concentration. In stages one, two, and three, there's no increase in concentration, even though the individual has a very low creatinine clearance. Generally, if you have a person with creatinine clearance above 30, there's no problem with magnesium supplementation. And, of course, we know who is in stages four and five, since they are already on dialysis. When someone is on dialysis, it's important to be extremely careful not to give magnesium without the oversight of a nephrologist. Having said this, for most of us magnesium is completely safe.

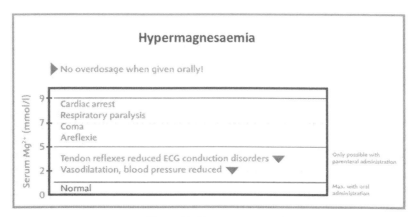

Figure 44: Hypermagnesaemia

If a person experiences hypermagnesaemia, which is too much magnesium in the blood—such as up to 4 mmol per litre—there are effects, but these can only be triggered by mistakes in the administration of intravenous infusion of magnesium, never by oral administration. Such effects can take the form of areflexia (a lack of reflexes), respiratory paralysis, cardiac arrest, and coma. We would see the tendon reflexes reduced, ECG conduction disorders, and vasodilation resulting in reduced blood pressure.

When there is too much magnesium from oral administration, the surplus is excreted through the kidneys, which is a relatively easy task. In fact, it's more complicated for the kidney not to excrete the excess of magnesium. Even with supplementation of 1,000 or more milligrams, it's not possible to achieve more than 1.2 mmol per litre of blood.

[27]

Do You Have
a Magnesium Deficiency?

How can you assess your magnesium status?

In the United States, Ronald J. Elin has done a lot of investigation of magnesium status utilising methods employed in clinical chemistry (Elin, 2010). For instance, we can measure total serum magnesium concentration. We can also measure the serum ionised concentration, though this is a little more complicated. Additionally, we can use a 24-hour urine excretion method. But by far the easiest measurement to make is total serum concentration. An evidence-based reference interval for serum magnesium concentration has been established, where the lower limit is adjusted to a value that's healthy, which is 0.85 mmol per litre.

It's important to realise that a concentration above this figure still doesn't exclude magnesium deficiency, since the blood sampling procedure itself can sometimes induce a magnesium loss from the cells. This occurs because some people are anxious about having a needle inserted into their arm, and stress drives magnesium out of the cells. ATP is broken down, and bound magnesium is released and transported out of the cells, ending up in the plasma. So stress produces an artificial increase in our magnesium plasma concentration. Consequently, a person may have a serum magnesium concentration of 0.9 mmol per litre, which on the surface looks like they have no problem with a magnesium deficiency.

What this amounts to is that the serum concentration of magnesium is indicative when it's low, but it doesn't tell us anything if our levels appear normal or above normal. In fact, a study (Ismail et al., 2010) advises that a health warning is needed for when there are "normal" results. This is to address the underestimated problem of using serum magnesium measurements to exclude magnesium deficiency in adults.

We want to quote from the conclusions of this study, because the information is so important. The authors state, "The inaccuracy of serum magnesium as a biomarker of negative body stores, although well known among laboratorians, is not widely disseminated nor emphasised to clinicians. The perception that 'normal' serum magnesium excludes deficiency is not uncommon among clinicians, and this has contributed to underdiagnosis of chronic deficiency. Based on literature in the last two decades, magnesium deficiency remains common and undervalued, warranting a proactive approach by the laboratory because restoration of magnesium stores is simple, tolerable, inexpensive and can be clinically beneficial."

In addition to identifying low serum magnesium concentrations, it's important to observe clinical symptoms. As mentioned earlier, these can include such things as cardiac arrhythmia, cramps, migraine, and headaches. It's also important to identify risk factors for low magnesium intake by asking such questions as what the person eats and whether there are factors such as increased loss of magnesium—for instance, from use of a diuretic or a protein pump inhibitor. The simple reality is that a large percentage of people need magnesium supplementation.

[28]

How to Select the Best Magnesium Supplement

Which magnesium salt should be used for supplementation?

Studies have shown the superior efficacy of magnesium citrate, when compared for instance with amino acid chelate or magnesium oxide (Walker et al., 2003). When all three forms were administered at the same dosage, only magnesium citrate increased the magnesium plasma concentration. This was true both in a 24-hour study and in a 60-day study, both of which supplemented with 300 milligrams of magnesium.

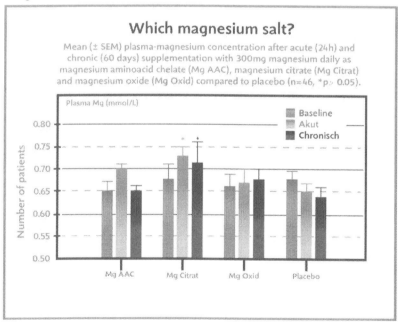

Figure 45: Which magnesium salt?

In another study using 600 milligrams of magnesium citrate, there was a significant advantage as the hours passed (Wilimzig et al., 1996). In fact, serum magnesium levels increased for a period of twelve hours. In the placebo group, we see only the effects of the circadian rhythm, whereby magnesium levels are naturally lower in the morning but increase as the day goes on, reaching a peak in the evening. The time to give magnesium is therefore at night. We don't understand precisely why magnesium levels drop during the night, causing them to be low by morning, but suspect it has something to do with kidney function and hormone regulation.

This drop in plasma concentrations correlates with clinical symptoms. When do people tend to get leg cramps? Mostly at night and early in the morning. When do we tend to see myocardial infarction? There is a peak in the early morning hours. Arrhythmia also tends to occur at night. Such symptoms can be avoided simply by giving magnesium in the evening. One effect of the elevation and leveling out of plasma magnesium levels that this results in is that people sleep better because they are more relaxed. Incidentally, taken as a tablet, magnesium citrate isn't as effective, since it needs to be pre-dissolved to obtain the most value from it.

You might wonder whether you should take magnesium at the same time as calcium. The answer is an emphatic "no." If you put calcium and magnesium together, such as in pill form, the high magnesium inhibits the calcium uptake, and the high calcium inhibits the magnesium uptake. If calcium supplementation is necessary, there needs to be a period of several hours between ingesting the magnesium and the calcium. For example, you could take calcium in the morning and magnesium in the evening. Having said this, a normal diet usually contains adequate calcium for the average person in acid-base balance, so that there's no requirement for supplementation.

Of even greater significance in terms of the effect of the kind of magnesium on the plasma magnesium concentration is the effect on the intracellular free magnesium concentration in human leukocytes. When we supplement with magnesium oxide, there's only a small effect on the intracellular free magnesium concentration in the leukocytes, whereas there's a much larger effect when we use the citrate form (Nestler et al., 2012). This is particularly significant because leukocytes are our immune cells, and a study published in Science in July 2013 shows that the level of magnesium in these cells is extremely important if they are to function effectively (Chaigne-Delalande et al., 2013). Magnesium regulates the cytotoxic function of natural killer cells in patients with a defect in the MAGT1 transporter. This was also mentioned in the journal Nature, meaning that the significance of magnesium is now a serious matter for science.

Magnesium regulates antiviral immunity. The latest findings reveal the specific molecular function of free basal intracellular magnesium in eukaryotic cells. It's the intracellular free magnesium concentration in lymphocytes that's important, and we can show that with magnesium citrate we get a much better uptake than with magnesium oxide. Because of its impact on our immunity, magnesium deficiency has a truly negative effect and should be avoided.

We need to point out that this difference isn't something we can measure on a routine basis in everyday practice, since it's a complicated procedure requiring a magnesium-sensitive dye to load the cells—a process that takes quite a while. From such protocols, we know that only those who have a low magnesium plasma concentration register a major change, whereas those whose level are at or above 0.85 experience no change at all. However, we must emphasise that we find this increase not with magnesium oxide, only with magnesium citrate. A person with a relatively normal plasma concentration who would like to increase their level needs to use citrate. Since citrate is readily available, we might mention that it's highly desirable to have a plasma concentration that's as high as possible, since (as discussed earlier) this provides protection against sudden cardiac death, diabetes, and so on.

The point we are making about using citrate instead of other forms of magnesium is further borne out by the case of a child born with an error in the ability to reabsorb magnesium in the kidneys (Bircan et al., 2006). The child developed severe cramps shortly after birth and was lucky to have a doctor who knew the importance of magnesium. Since this was a case of primary hypomagnesaemia, it was initially treated intravenously. However, such treatment is neither practical nor desirable on a daily basis, so the child was then supplemented with the various forms of magnesium that are available. Those handling the case discovered that only with magnesium citrate were they able to establish the extremely high dose needed by the child—a dosage of 88 milligrams per kilogram of body weight. For a child weighing 20 kilograms, that's around 1,900 milligrams on a daily basis! Today, the child is still on the high dose of magnesium citrate and, at twelve or thirteen years of age, is symptom free.

What about other magnesium compounds, such as magnesium orotate? The problem with this form is that the actual amount of magnesium delivered is relatively low. Unfortunately, many preparations that contain this form don't state how much magnesium is supplied, only how much magnesium orotate is present. In such a case, you might get 500 milligrams of magnesium orotate, but only something like 30 milligrams of magnesium. Do you really want to take twenty tablets a day to get 600 milligrams?

Magnesium is only absorbed as an ion, not as a complex. Were it absorbed as a complex, the child discussed earlier could easily be treated with a substance such as magnesium bisglycinate, which is claimed to be is absorbed as a peptide. When magnesium is bound to something, it simply isn't absorbed. So it's not much better then magnesium oxide. The crucial issue with any supplement is an understanding of how it's transported into the cells.

When you are purchasing a magnesium product, be aware that just because something says "magnesium" doesn't mean it's useful to the body, since there are a number of factors involved in the absorption of the mineral. In its citrate form, it does the job—and you can take it lifelong. Professor Vormann has been taking it for more than 30 years.

Were magnesium absorbed into the cells through the skin, such as in the form magnesium oil, all we would need to do is go swimming in the ocean, since the ocean is high in magnesium. But magnesium isn't absorbed this way—although the oil can be used topically for certain skin diseases. The skin is nearly impermeable in the case of both magnesium and calcium. The genes now known to be involved in magnesium uptake only use magnesium ions, not complexes. A wise decision therefore is to use magnesium citrate.

[29]

Conclusion

Even as earth's inhabitants migrated out of the original cradle of humanity, spreading out across the planet and colonising continent after continent, so too the landmasses, we now inhabit as a species, have themselves shifted over eons of time. Land that was once submerged now forms mountains, while mountains were once the ocean floor. Vast regions have come into existence as a result of plate tectonics and volcanic activity that never existed before.

As humans spread out around the world, they encountered different climates producing different foodstuffs. Seasons came into play in a way they never had where our species had its nativity, hugely affecting the diet of our ancestors. Equally important, some of the younger soils produced not only different kinds but also different qualities of foods, since all growing media are not the same. Some zones were rich in one mineral but not in another, one nutrient but not another. Also, in more recent times, modern farming methods have depleted soils in vast areas.

Today, we aren't often aware of how greatly the nutrients in our food supply vary according to how, where, and when the food was grown. With planes jetting fresh fruits to parts of the globe that don't naturally produce such fruit, an abundance of meats, and boatloads of foodstuffs shipped all over the world, it's easy to think of a Paleo diet in terms of the foods advocated for such a diet by books and websites that have made this their trademark. In reality, a Paleo diet consumed by our ancestors was considerably different from what we think of when we use this term today.

Yet there is a commonality among all these diets—their tendency to alkalinity and an abundance of health-giving organic minerals. Even when we do our best to eat a balanced diet, in our modern world, we tend to short-change ourselves when it comes to alkalinity and minerals, such as magnesium.

The modern health-conscious individual is wise to select as alkalising a diet as is practical, without neglecting an adequate supply of protein. Supplementation, especially when done under the supervision of a medical professional who is aware of the emerging science in the field, is a potent method of optimising our health on many levels.

Never before has the science been available to guide us in ridding ourselves of the scourge of magnesium-poor and acid-rich diets. As the facts become increasingly available, it's time for all of us, young and old, to take advantage of what we now know—and begin to experience a quality of life we didn't imagine possible, particularly as we age.

Appendix 1

For a very quick magnesium status indication, it is recommended to go to: *www.magnesiumguide.com.au/magnesium-minute/*

1. Magnesium Dietary Depleter – issue with magnesium intake.

Description: A magnesium dietary depleter tends to have a diet lacking in whole grains, green vegetables, and legumes. According to a CSIRO study, approximately 50% of Australian men and 39% of Australian women are not getting sufficient magnesium in their diet. Such individuals respond well to both dietary changes and supplementation. It should be noted that absorption rises when dietary intake is low and drops when dietary intake, including supplements, is high. For example, a normal absorption rate for magnesium is 30-50%, though this can rise to 80% if intake is very low.

Assessment: You may be a magnesium dietary depleter if you complete the assessment in Table 1 with a score of less than 20.

Assessment Tools:

- Magnesium Dietary Depleter Assessment Table 1
- Blood tests may or may not indicate deficiency, depending on severity
- Plasma magnesium – low or on low side of normal
- Urinary magnesium – low or on low side of normal.

Solutions

Dietary/Lifestyle: Increase dietary sources of magnesium. Increase consumption of organic wholegrains, green vegetables and legumes in the diet. Use the 'Magnesium Rich Foods' list available from Bio-Practica.
Supplementation: Supplement with a highly bioavailable, clinically trialled magnesium. One sachet per day. Adjust dosing amount for children younger than 12 years.

Table 1. Magnesium Dietary Depleter Assesment

How many times per week do you [does your patient] consume the following foods

Food	Almost everyday or everyday	Regularly (2-5 times per week)	Sometimes (once or less per week)	Rarely or never
Adzuki beans	3	2	1	0
Almonds (unsalted)	3	2	1	0
Baby beetroot leaves	3	2	1	0
Black-eyed peas	3	2	1	0
Beet greens	3	2	1	0
Brazil nuts (unsalted)	3	2	1	0
Brown rice	3	2	1	0
Buckwheat	3	2	1	0
Cashews (unsalted)	3	2	1	0
Figs	3	2	1	0
Halibut (fish)	3	2	1	0
Hazelnuts (unsalted)	3	2	1	0
Kelp	3	2	1	0
Kidney beans	3	2	1	0
Lentils	3	2	1	0
Linseeds	3	2	1	0
Low fat yoghurt	3	2	1	0
Macadamia nuts (unsalted)	3	2	1	0
Mixed lettuce greens (rocket, mesclun, endive, arugula, dandelion etc)	3	2	1	0
Millet	3	2	1	0
Oatmeal	3	2	1	0
Pecans (unsalted)	3	2	1	0
Pistachios	3	2	1	0
Pumpkin seeds	3	2	1	0
Rice bran/Oat bran/Wheat bran	3	2	1	0
Sesame seeds	3	2	1	0
Soy beans	3	2	1	0
Spinach or baby spinach	3	2	1	0
Spirulina	3	2	1	0
Sunflower seeds	3	2	1	0
Walnuts	3	2	1	0
SECTION 1. TOTAL SCORE				

A score less the 20 indicates a 'Dietary Depleter Type'   'Dietary Depleter Type' Yes ☐   No ☐

119

2. Magnesium Malabsorber – Intestinal issue

Description: Magnesium malabsorbers may be taking supplements and still not get results, or they may have to take higher than expected supplementation to produce results. Factors, such as ageing, poor digestion, high calcium levels, toxicity and diarrhoea can lead to ineffective absorption of magnesium. It is critical to supplement with a magnesium supplement that is well absorbed.

Assessment: The individual may experience symptoms of magnesium deficiency along with malabsorption issues such as nausea, vomiting, bloating, muscle wasting, unexplained weight loss, abdominal pain or cramping, bulky stools, steatorrhea, undigested food in stool, and so on.

Assessment Tools:

- Magnesium Malabsorber checklist Table 2
- Practitioner Magnesium Malabsorber checklist
- Blood tests may or may not indicate deficiency, depending on severity
- Plasma magnesium – low or low side of normal
- Urinary magnesium – low or low side of normal
- RBC (red blood cell) magnesium (Reference range: 1.70-2.80 mmol/L).

A number of health conditions automatically indicate issues with magnesium absorption, including primary infantile hypomagnesaemia, ulcerative colitis, Whipple's disease, short bowel syndrome, intestinal resection, and Crohn's disease.

Solutions

Dietary/Lifestyle: Address absorption issues. In general, the degree of magnesium depletion correlates with the severity of diarrhoea, stool fat content, and faecal magnesium concentration. The malabsorption of magnesium is secondary to the formation of insoluble magnesium soaps, and a low fat diet improves magnesium balance in these patients.

Other suggestions:

1. Repair and nourish the digestive tract using therapeutic agents, such as glutamine and probiotics.
2. Calm and improve digestion with ginger, lemon juice and water.
3. Add slippery elm powder to the diet and cook with curcumin, ginger and dill to reduce inflammation and irritation to the gut lining.
4. Stop to eat, eat slowly, and chew well to ensure stimulation of natural digestion.
5. Reduce dietary phytates, oxalates, phosphorus and potassium, if excessive, as they reduce magnesium absorption.

Supplementation:

- Highly bioavailable, clinically trialled magnesium in a large bottle of water. Drink throughout the day to maximise absorption. Adjust dosing amount for children younger than 12 years.
- Highly bioavailable curcumin extract to help reduce inflammation of the gastrointestinal tract.
- High strength multi strain probiotic to support healthy gut microflora.
- Gut healing formulations/support programs should be considered.

Genetics: Inherited mutation in the TRPM 6 gene – codes for an ion channel, resulting in defective carrier mediated transport of Mg in the small intestine. Absorption reduced from 70% to 35%. The defect can be overcome by increasing oral intake of magnesium to approximately 5 times that of normal daily requirements. Presents with hypocalcaemia, tetany, and seizures.

Table 2. Check list for Magnesium Malabsorber:

Signs and Symptoms
- 5 or more of the following signs and symptoms indicates a Mg Malabsorber type

Burps after meals regularly	☐
Heartburn regularly	☐
Flatulence regularly	☐
Bad breath regularly	☐
Takes Iron or Zinc supplements regularly without Magnesium	☐
Takes Calcium supplements without Magnesium	☐
Is over 50 years of age	☐
Regularly supplements their diet with protein powder (everyday)	☐
Eats a diet very high in protein (fish, chicken, eggs, meat) every day	☐
Has loose stools or diarrhoea 3 or more times per week	☐
Consumes a diet high in dairy products (more than 3 serves per day)	☐
Consumes a diet high in fatty foods daily (fried foods, butter, hamburgers, bacon, ice-cream, cheese, oils)	☐
Frequently has undigested food or fat in their stools (more than 3 times per week)	☐
Frequently uses antibiotics (more than 3 courses in the last 6 months)	☐
Has known low vitamin B1 levels	☐
Has known low vitamin D levels	☐
Has known low Vitamin B6 levels	☐
Has known high 'heavy metal' levels (Mercury, Cadmium, Lead, Aluminium, Arsenic)	☐
Has high 'Insulin' levels	☐
Has recent or known parasites or worms	☐
Steatorrhoea (excessive fats in the stool)	☐
Has unexplained weight loss	☐
Experiences abdominal pain or cramping	☐
Has some degree of intestinal permeability	☐

Known health conditions
- One or more of the following indications an Mg Malabsorber type

Irritable Bowel Syndrome (IBS)	☐
Hypoparathyroidism	☐
Crohn's disease	☐
Bulimia	☐
Ulcerative colitis	☐
Celiac disease	☐
Whipples disease	☐
Multiple Sclerosis	☐
Known genetic disorders affecting absorption (eg. TRPM 6 gene)	☐
Had intestinal resection	☐
Short Bowel Syndrome	☐
Medically diagnosed malnutrition	☐
Diabetes	☐

'Magnesium Malabsorber Type' Yes ☐ No ☐

3. Magnesium Hyper-excreter – issue with kidneys

Description: Hyper-excreters eliminate excessive amounts of magnesium through the kidneys and urine. They often have normal levels of magnesium in blood tests, but what we are actually seeing is higher levels of magnesium being excreted and very little retained in the body. They will often have increased magnesium in the urine. It is critical to supplement with a magnesium supplement that gets into the cells, and address the issues that may be causing excessive excretion, which can be dietary, drugs, kidney disorders, and so on.

Assessment: The individual may manifest symptoms of magnesium deficiency along with excretion issues such as kidney disorders, phosphate depletion, acidity, hypercalcaemia, and hormonal issues (PTH, calcitonin, antidiuretic hormone).

Assessment Tools:

- Magnesium Hyper-excreter checklist Table 3
- Blood Tests: Magnesium may or may not be low depending on level of deficiency
- Plasma Magnesium – low or normal
- Urinary Magnesium – generally high or high side of normal.
- RBC Magnesium – (Reference range: 1.70-2.80 mmol/L)

A number of health conditions may automatically indicate excretion issues, such as Barters syndrome, Gitelman's syndrome, primary hyperparathyroidism, malignant hypercalcaemia, hyperthyroidism, hyperaldosteronism, diabetes, etc.

Drugs, such as diuretics, cytotoxic drugs (cisplatin, carboplatin, gallium nitrate), antimicrobial agents (aminoglycosides, antituberculous drugs, immunosuppressants), beta adrenergic agonists, amphotericin B, pentamidine, foscarnet, pamidronate, anascrin.

Osmotic diuretics, such as mannitol and glucose, cause marked increase in magnesium excretion.
(R Swaminathan, Magnesium Metabolism and its Disorders. Clin Biochem Rev. 2003 May; 24(2): 47–66).

Solutions

Dietary/Lifestyle: It is essential to reduce stress exposure, practice meditation and make the following dietary changes to avoid triggering excess excretion:

1. Reduce or avoid mannitol and glucose in the diet
2. Minimise carbonated drinks (fizzy drinks)
3. Reduce or avoid tea and coffee
4. Reduce or avoid alcohol
5. Ensure you are drinking adequate water daily (8-10 glasses)

Supplementation:
- Highly bioavailable, clinically trialled magnesium: 1-2 sachets per day, depending on severity of deficiency. Adjust dosing for children under 12 years.
- Comprehensive Lymphatic Support Formula: To support kidney health.
- Herbal calming formula: To reduce stress and the associated hormonal changes.

Table 3. Magnesium Hyper-excreter check list:

Consumes soft drinks / fizzy drinks daily	☐
Drinks 3 or more cups of coffee per day	☐
Drinks up to 5 cups of tea per day	☐
Consumes high sugar containing foods daily (chocolate, candy, lollies, ice-cream, cakes, biscuits, donuts etc.)	☐
Consumes fruit juice drinks everyday (two or more glasses of fruit juice per day)	☐
Lives or works in a high stress environment or is currently stressed	☐
Drinks alcohol everyday or more than 7 alcoholic drinks per week	☐
Does strenuous exercise or training more than 3 times per week (running, sports, gym etc)	☐
Experiences excessive sweating (more than 3 times per week)	☐
Takes steroid medication (e.g. Prednisolone, Symbacort, Cortisone)	☐
Takes Digitalis (Digoxin – a heart medication)	☐
Takes any of the following medication: Foscarnet (anti-viral drug), Amphotericin B (anti-fungal drug), Cyclosporin (immunosuppressant drug), Azathioprine (immunosuppressant drug), Crisplatin (chemotherapy drug).	☐
Has low Selenium levels	☐
Has high Calcium levels	☐
Has acid/alkali imbalance	☐
Has high Vitamin D	☐
Has high Potassium levels	☐
Has high blood pressure	☐
Has high Insulin levels	☐
Is often dehydrated (does not drink enough water)	☐

Known health conditions
- One or more of the following indications a Mg Hyper-excreter type

Alcoholism	☐
Chronic kidney disease (kidney failure, Dialysis)	☐
Genetic kidney disorder (eg. Barters syndrome, Gitelman syndrome)	☐
Diabetes	☐
Diabetic nephropathy	☐
Takes any kind of diuretic medication (Thiazides, Osmotic diuretics, Loop diuretics etc.)	☐
Nephritis	☐
Renal fibrosis	☐
Kidney stones	☐
Hyperparathyroidism	☐
Hyperaldosteronism	☐
Hyperthyroidism	☐
Hypocalcaemia	☐
Recurrent cystitis	☐
Recurrent kidney infections	☐

'Magnesium Hyper-excreter Type'   Yes ☐   No ☐

125

Magnesium Demander – metabolic issue

Description: The magnesium demander has an increased need for magnesium due to certain lifestyle factors. Those with increased demand include pregnant/lactating women, athletes, growing children, stressed individuals, and the ageing.

Assessment: The individual may or may not initially manifest many symptoms of magnesium deficiency, but may have a health issue or condition that increases their body's metabolic need for magnesium.

Assessment Tools:
Magnesium Demander Checklist Table 4

Solutions

Dietary/Lifestyle: Reduce stress and increase dietary intake of magnesium food groups.

Supplementation:
- Highly bioavailable, clinically trialled magnesium: 1-2 sachets daily. Adjust dosing for children under 12 years.
- Energy/Thyroid formula and or herbal calming formula for highly stressed individuals.
- Clinically trialled alkalising mineral drink for athletes and high intensity exercise.

Table 4. Magnesium Demander check list:

Currently pregnant	☐
Recently pregnant (in the last 12 months)	☐
Breastfeeding or recently breastfed for longer than 12 months	☐
Recent traumatic stress, physical or emotional (in the last 6 months)	☐
Lives or works in a stressful environment or is currently stressed	☐
PMS or menstrual cramps	☐
Chronic lethargy or fatigue	☐
Has trouble sleeping most nights (more than 3 nights per week)	☐
Drinks alcohol everyday or more than 7 alcoholic drinks per week	☐
Over 50 years of age	☐
Strenuous exercise or training more than 3 times per week (running, sports, gym etc)	☐

Known health conditions
– One or more of the following indicates an Mg Demander Type

Insomnia	☐
Cardiovascular disease (Arrhythmia, Atherosclerosis, congestive heart failure or recent cardiovascular 'event').	☐
High blood pressure	☐
Recent pancreatitis	☐
Recent blood transfusion	☐
Recent saline infusion	☐
Fibromyalgia	☐
Diabetes (insulin dependent)	☐
Osteoporosis	☐
PTSD (post traumatic stress disorder)	☐
Asthma	☐
An overactive thyroid, or underactive thyroid	☐
Depression	☐
Glaucoma	☐
Chronic headaches or migraines	☐
An endocrine condition such as Hyperaldosteronism or Hyperparathyroidism	☐
Have diagnosed Haemochromatosis (Iron overload)	☐
In a previous pregnancy had high blood pressure or preeclampsia	☐
Taking oral contraceptives	☐
Recent severe burns	☐

'Magnesium Demander Type'   Yes ☐   No ☐

127

5. Magnesium Multi-depleter

Description: Any combination of low dietary intake, absorption, demand, and/or excretion issues. Such individuals often require magnesium supplementation as well as have their multiple underlying issues addressed, according to which magnesium type issues they have. Having multiple depletion issues, magnesium status and underlying issues should be treated with high priority.

Assessment: The individual may evidence any of the above signs and symptoms of magnesium deficiency and/or known health conditions in any type.

Assessment Tools:

- Plasma Magnesium – low
- Urinary Magnesium – low or high, depending on their types
- RBC Magnesium – (Reference range: 1.70-2.80 mmol/L)

Solutions

Dietary/Lifestyle: Treat as for each individual type, as it presents. For example, an individual may present as multi-depleter; hyper-excreter/demander. Then treat as per these sections suggest.

Supplementation:

Highly bioavailable, clinically trialled magnesium: 1-2 sachets daily. Adjust dosing for children under 12 years.

APPENDIX 2:
YOUTUBE VIDEO RESOURCES:

MAGNESIUM DEFICIENCY QUESTIONS ANSWERED
BY PROFESSOR VORMANN:

Question 1: What are the factors to consider when selecting a Magnesium Supplement? http://youtu.be/4RajrL8XMnM

Question 2: Which is best? Magnesium Tablet Vs Magnesium Powder: http://youtu.be/IbysEB2Zvw8

Question 3: What is your opinion of Multi Ingredient Magnesium Supplements? http://youtu.be/pPPCmx39hjQ

Question 4: Is Magnesium Citrate the best form of magnesium? http://youtu.be/zns3rr-ujXw

Question 5: Is Magnesium Citrate the best form of magnesium? Long Answer. http://youtu.be/nzqpiI7A7Es

Question 6: Is it true that magnesium can be absorbed as a complex molecule? http://youtu.be/z-V0RbILlio

Question 7: Do we get enough magnesium in our diet? http://youtu.be/_suUZzshxE0

Question 8: Is there a magnesium deficiency crisis? Why? http://youtu.be/8yknNBC8azQ

Question 9: Can we deplete our magnesium Levels? http://youtu.be/vk-lQGjF8hA

Question 10: Why are high doses of magnesium required? http://youtu.be/5ww7Pre586s

Question 11: Are there disease states that respond to high doses of magnesium? http://youtu.be/__RosCSP2UE

Question 12: Is there interesting research of the relationship of magnesium status and diabetes? http://youtu.be/t2RxSsJdxdU

Question 13: How do you know how much available magnesium is in a supplement? http://youtu.be/u4KbqinKLJA

Question 14: Why is magnesium essential during pregnancy? http://youtu.be/CCEb1-u1fN0

Question 15: Why is magnesium essential during stress? http://youtu.be/AyqYWXDlRiU

Question 16: After 30 years of research into magnesium in your opinion how important is magnesium to health? http://youtu.be/PbkFRJPOeFQ

Question 17: When is the best time to take magnesium? http://youtu.be/POUOgFFuhWk

Question 18: What is the relationship of magnesium status and sudden cardiac death? http://youtu.be/IWR-QmS7eo8

Question 19: What does the research tell us about magnesium status and cardiac disease? http://youtu.be/Tf8YPUHxpUw

Bibliography

Adeva MM, Souto G. Diet-induced metabolic acidosis. Clin Nutr. 2011 ;30:416-21, 2011

Akter S, Eguchi M, Kuwahara K, Kochi T, Ito R, Kurotani K, Tsuruoka H, Nanri A, Kabe I, Mizoue T. High dietary acid load is associated with insulin resistance: The Furukawa Nutrition and Health Study. Clin Nutr. S0261-5614, 2015

Alexy U, Remer T, Manz F, Neu CM , Schoenau E. Long-term protein intake and dietary potential renal acid load are associated with bone modeling and remodeling at the proximal radius in healthy children. Am J Clin Nutr. 82, 1107-1114, 2005.

Atwood CS, Moir RD, Huang X, Scarpa RC, Bacarra NM, Romano DM, Hartshorn MA, Tanzi RE, Bush AI.Dramatic aggregation of Alzheimer abeta by Cu(II) is induced by conditions representing physiological acidosis. J Biol Chem. 273:12817-26, 1998.

Australian Health Survey: Usual Nutrient Intakes, 2011-12, www.abs.gov.au, 2015

Aydin H, Deyneli O, Yavuz D, Gözü H, Mutlu N, Kaygusuz I, Akalin S. Short-term oral magnesium supplementation suppresses bone turnover in postmenopausal osteoporotic women. Biol Trace Elem Res. 2010:133:136-43.

Barbagallo M, Belvedere M, Di Bella G, Dominguez LJ. Mg is reduced in mild-to-moderate Alzheimer's disease. Magnes Res. 24:115-21, 2011

Barbagallo M, Dominguez LJ, Galioto A, Pineo A, Belvedere M. Oral magnesium supplementation improves vascular function in elderly diabetic patients. Magnes Res. 23:131-7, 2010

Barragán-Rodríguez L, Rodríguez-Morán M, Guerrero-Romero F. Efficacy and safety of oral magnesium supplementation in the treatment of depression in the elderly with type 2 diabetes: a randomized, equivalent trial. Magnes Res. 21:218-23, 2008

Berkemeyer S, Vormann J, Günther AL, Rylander R, Frassetto LA, Remer T. Renal net acid excretion capacity is comparable in prepubescence, adolescence, and young adulthood but falls with aging. J Am Geriatr Soc. 56:1442-8, 2008.

Bircan I, Turkkahraman D, Dursun O, Karaguzel G. Successful management of primary hypomagnesaemia with high-dose oral magnesium citrate: a case report. Acta Paediatr. 95:1697-9, 2006

Boschmann M, Michalsen A, Kaiser N, Meier L, Stange R. Acid-base balance and local muscular metabolism of healthy elderly during protein-rich diet with or without alkaline supplements. International Congress on Integrative Medicine and Health. Las Vegas, USA, 2016

Buclin T, Cosma M, Appenzeller M, Jacquet AF, Décosterd LA, Biollaz J, Burckhardt P. Diet acids and alkalis influence calcium retention in bone. Osteoporos Int. 12:493- 9, 2001

Bullarbo M, Ödman N, Nestler A, Nielsen T, Kolisek M, Vormann J, Rylander R. Magnesium supplementation to prevent high blood pressure in pregnancy: a randomised placebo control trial. Arch Gynecol Obstet. 288:1269-74, 2013

Chaigne-Delalande B, Li FY, O'Connor GM, Lukacs MJ, Jiang P, Zheng L, Shatzer A, Biancalana M, Pittaluga S, Matthews HF, Jancel TJ, Bleesing JJ, Marsh RA, Kuijpers TW, Nichols KE, Lucas CL, Nagpal S, Mehmet H, Su HC, Cohen JI, Uzel G, Lenardo MJ. Mg2+ regulates cytotoxic functions of NK and CD8 T cells in chronic EBV infection through NKG2D. Science 341:186-91, 2013

Chiuve SE, Korngold EC, Januzzi JL Jr, Gantzer ML, Albert CM. Plasma and dietary magnesium and risk of sudden cardiac death in women. Am J Clin Nutr. 93:253-60, 2011

Chiuve SE, Sun Q, Curhan GC, Taylor EN, Spiegelman D, Willett WC, Manson JE, Rexrode KM, Albert CM. Dietary and plasma magnesium and risk of coronary heart disease among women. J Am Heart Assoc. 18; 2:e000114, 2013

Cilliler AE1, Ozturk S, Ozbakir S. Low serum magnesium level correlates to clinical deterioration in Alzheimer's disease. Gerontology 53:419-22, 2007

Coburn JW, Popovtzer MM, Massry SG, Kleeman CR. The physicochemical state and renal handling of divalent ions in chronic renal failure. Arch Intern Med. 124:302-11, 1969

Cordain L, Eaton SB, Sebastian A, Mann N, Lindeberg S, Watkins BA, O'Keefe JH, Brand-Miller J. Origins and evolution of the Western diet: health implications for the 21st century. Am J Clin Nutr 81: 341-54, 2005.

Cseuz R, Barna I, Bender T, Vormann J. Alkaline Mineral Supplementation Decreases Pain in Rheumatoid Arthritis Patients: A Pilot Study. The Open Nutrition Journal 2, 100-105, 2008.

de Baaij JH, Hoenderop JG, Bindels RJ. Magnesium in man: implications for health and disease. Physiol Rev. 95:1-46, 2015

Dong JY, Xun P, He K, Qin LQ. Magnesium intake and risk of type 2 diabetes: meta-analysis of prospective cohort studies. Diabetes Care 34:2116-22, 2011

Edited by Robert Vink, University Adelaide Press, pp 115-124, 2011

Elin RJ. Assessment of magnesium status for diagnosis and therapy. Magnes Res. 23:194-8. 2010

Etulain J, Negrotto S, Carestia A, Pozner RG, Romaniuk MA, D'Atri LP, Klement GL, Schattner M. Acidosis downregulates platelet haemostatic functions and promotes neutrophil proinflammatory responses mediated by platelets. Thromb Haemost. 107:99-110, 2012.

Fagherazzi et al. Dietary acid load and risk of type 2 diabetes: the E3N-EPIC cohort study. Diabetologia. 2014 ;57:313-20, 2014

Farr M, Garvey K, Bold AM, Kendall MJ, Bacon PA. Significance of the hydrogen ion concentration in synovial fluid in rheumatoid arthritis. Clin Exp Rheumatol 3: 99-104, 1985.

Frassetto LA, Sebastian A. Age and systemic acid-base equilibrium: analysis of published data. J Gerontol A Biol Sci Med Sci. 51: B91-99, 1996.

Frassetto LA, Todd KM, Morris RC Jr., Sebastian A: Worldwide incidence of hip fracture in elderly women: relation to consumption of animal and vegetable foods. J Gerontol. 55A:M585-M592, 2000.

Frick KK, Bushinsky DA: Metabolic acidosis stimulates RANKL RNA expression in bone through a cyclo-oxygenase-dependent mechanism. J Bone Miner Res 18:1317-1325, 2003.

Frick KK, LaPlante K, Bushinsky DA. RANK ligand and TNF-alpha mediate acid-induced bone calcium efflux in vitro. Am J Physiol 289: F1005-10, 2005.

Grinspoon SK, Baum HB, Kim V, Coggins C, Klibanski A. Decreased bone formation and increased mineral dissolution during acute fasting in young women. J Clin Endocrinol Metab.80:3628-33, 1995

Guerrero-Romero et al. Oral magnesium supplementation improves insulin sensitivity in non-diabetic subjects with insulin resistance. A double-blind placebo-controlled randomized trial. Diabetes Metab. 30:253-8, 2004

Guerrero-Romero F, Rodríguez-Morán M. Hypomagnesemia, oxidative stress, inflammation, and metabolic syndrome. Diabetes Metab Res Rev. 22:471-6, 2006

Hashimoto T, Nishi K, Nagasao J, Tsuji S, Oyanagi K. Magnesium exerts both preventive and ameliorating effects in an in vitro rat Parkinson disease model. Brain Res. 1197:143-51, 2008

Hill J, Micklewright A, Lewis S, Britton J. Investigation of the effect of short-term change in dietary magnesium intake in asthma. Eur. Respiratory J.10:2225-2229, 1997

Hoane MR. The role of magnesium therapy in learning and memory. In: Magnesium in the Central Nervous System

Holzer P. Acid-sensitive ion channels and receptors. Handb Exp Pharmacol. 194:283-332, 2009

Hood VL, Tannen RL. Protection of acid-base balance by pH regulation of acid production. N Engl J Med. 1998;339:819-26

Hottenrott L, Meyer TP, Vormann J, Werner T, Hottenrott K. Effects of intermittent fasting combined with alkaline mineral supplementation and exercise training on weight loss. A 12 weeks placebo-controlled double-blind trial with overweight subjects. 21st Annual Congress of the European College of Sport Science, Vienna, Austria, 2016

Humpel C.Chronic mild cerebrovascular dysfunction as a cause for Alzheimer's disease? Exp Gerontol. 46:225-32, 2011.

Ismail Y, Ismail AA, Ismail AA. The underestimated problem of using serum magnesium measurements to exclude magnesium deficiency in adults; a health warning is needed for "normal" results. Clin Chem Lab Med. 48:323-7, 2010

Jehle S, Hulter HN, Krapf R. Effect of potassium citrate on bone density, microarchitecture, and fracture risk in healthy older adults without osteoporosis: a randomized controlled trial. J Clin Endocrinol Metab. 98:207-17, 2013.

Jehle S, Zanetti A, Muser J, Hulter HN, Krapf R. Partial neutralization of the acidogenic Western diet with potassium citrate increases bone mass in postmenopausal women with osteopenia. J Am Soc Nephrol. 17:3213-22, 2006.

Kazaks AG, Uriu-Adams JY, Albertson TE, Shenoy SF, Stern JS. Effect of oral magnesium supplementation on measures of airway resistance and subjective assessment of asthma control and quality of life in men and women with mild to moderate asthma: a randomized placebo controlled trial. J Asthma. 47:83-92, 2010

Kelly GS. Hydrochloric Acid: Physiological Functions and Clinical Implications Alt Med Rev 1997; 2:116-127Achlorhydria References Pete??

Kim DJ, Xun P, Liu K, Loria C, Yokota K, Jacobs DR Jr, He K. Magnesium intake in relation to systemic inflammation, insulin resistance, and the incidence of diabetes. Diabetes Care 33:2604-10, 2010

Kohlmeier et al. Versorgung Erwachsener mit Mineralstoffen und Spurenelementen in der Bundesrepublik Deutschland. In: Kübler, W., Andersen, H. J., Heeschen, W. (Hrsg.) Vera-Schriftenreihe Band V, Wissenschaftlicher Fachverlag Dr. Fleck, Niederkleen, 1995.

Kolisek M, Nestler A, Vormann J, Schweigel-Röntgen M. Human gene SLC41A1 encodes for the Na+/Mg^{2}+ exchanger. Am J Physiol Cell Physiol. 302:C318-26, 2012

Köseoglu E, Talaslioglu A, Gönül AS, Kula M. The effects of magnesium prophylaxis in migraine without aura. Magnes Res. 21:101-8, 2008

Lameris AL, Monnens LA, Bindels RJ, Hoenderop JG.. Drug-induced alterations in Mg2+ homoeostasis. Clin Sci. 123:1-14, 2012

Larsson SC, Orsini N, Wolk A. Dietary magnesium intake and risk of stroke: a meta-analysis of prospective studies. Am J Clin Nutr. 95:362-6, 2012

Larsson SC, Wolk A.. Magnesium intake and risk of type 2 diabetes: a meta-analysis. J Intern Med. 262:208-14, 2007

Lemann, J Jr, Litzow JR, Lennon EJ: The effects of chronic acid loads in normal man: Further evidence for the participation of bone mineral in the defense against chronic metabolic acidosis. J Clin Invest 45: 1608-1614, 1966.

Lodi R, Iotti S, Cortelli P, Pierangeli G, Cevoli S, Clementi V, Soriani S, Montagna P, Barbiroli B. Deficient energy metabolism is associated with low free magnesium in the brains of patients with migraine and cluster headache. Brain Res Bull. 54:437-41, 2001

Lopez-Ridaura R1, Willett WC, Rimm EB, Liu S, Stampfer MJ, Manson JE, Hu FB.. Magnesium intake and risk of type 2 diabetes in men and women. Diabetes Care 27:134-40, 2004

Lutz J. Calcium balance and acid–base status of women as affected by increased protein intake and by sodium bicarbonate ingestion. Am J Clin Nutr 39: 281-8, 1984.

Marangella M, Di Stefano M, Casalis S, Berutti S, D'Amelio P, Isaia GC. Effects of potassium citrate supplementation on bone metabolism. Calcif Tissue Int 74: 330-5, 2004.

Maurer M, Riesen W, Muser J, Hulter HN, Krapf R. Neutralization of Western diet inhibits bone resorption independently of K intake and reduces cortisol secretion in humans. Am J Physiol Renal Physiol. 284:F32-40, 2003.

Mauskop A, Varughese J. Why all migraine patients should be treated with magnesium. J Neural Transm. 119:575-9, 2012

May RC, Kelly RA, Mitch WE. Metabolic acidosis stimulates protein degradation in rat muscle by a glucocorticoid-dependent mechanism. J Clin Invest. 77:614-21, 1986.

McCarty MF. Acid-base balance may influence risk for insulin resistance syndrome by modulating cortisol output. Med Hypotheses. 64:380-4, 2005.

Nationale Verzehrs Studie II, Max Rubner Institut, BFEL, 2008

Nestler A, Vormann J, Kolisek M. Magnesium Supplementation acutely affects intracellular Mg2+ in Human Leukocytes. The FASEB Journal 26:lb278, 2012

New SA, MacDonald HM, Campbell MK, Martin JC, Garton MJ, Robins SP, Reid DM. Lower estimates of net endogenous non-carbonic acid production are positively associated with indexes of bone health in premenopausal and perimenopausal women. Am J Clin Nutr 79: 131-8, 2004.

Nielsen FH, Milne DB, Klevay LM, Gallagher S, Johnson L.Dietary magnesium deficiency induces heart rhythm changes, impairs glucose tolerance, and decreases serum cholesterol in post menopausal women. J Am Coll Nutr. 26:121-32. 2007

Otsuki et al.. Association of urine acidification with visceral obesity and the metabolic syndrome. Endocr J. 2011;58:363-7, 2011

Peikert A, Wilimzig C, Köhne-Volland R. Prophylaxis of migraine with oral magnesium: results from a prospective, multi-center, placebo-controlled and double-blind randomized study. Cephalalgia 16:257-63, 1996

Pizzorno J, Frassetto LA, Katzinger J. Diet-induced acidosis: is it real and clinically relevant? Br J Nutr. 103:1185-94, 2010.

Qu X, Jin F, Hao Y, Li H, Tang T, Wang H, Yan W, Dai K. Magnesium and the Risk of Cardiovascular Events: A Meta-Analysis of Prospective Cohort Studies. PLoS ONE 8: e57720, 2013

Rae C, Scott RB, Thompson CH, Kemp GJ, Dumughn I, Styles P, Tracey I, Radda GK. Is pH a biochemical marker of IQ? Proc Biol Sci. 263:1061-4,1996.

Reddy ST, Wang CY, Sakhaee K, Brinkley L, Pak CY. Effect of low-carbohydrate high-protein diets on acid-base balance, stone-forming propensity, and calcium metabolism. Am J Kidney Dis 40:265-74, 2002.

Reffelmann T, Ittermann T, Dörr M, Völzke H, Reinthaler M, Petersmann A, Felix SB. Low serum magnesium concentrations predict cardiovascular and all-cause mortality. Atherosclerosis 219:280-4, 2011

Remer T, Manz F. Potential renal acid load (PRAL) of foods and its influence on urine pH. Am Diet Assoc 95: 791-7, 1995.

Robey IF, Martin NK. Bicarbonate and dichloroacetate: evaluating pH altering therapies in a mouse model for metastatic breast cancer. BMC Cancer 11:235, 2011

Rylander R, Remer T, Berkemeyer S, Vormann J. Acid-base status affects renal magnesium losses in healthy, elderly persons. J Nutr. 136: 2374-7, 2006.

Sebastian A, Frassetto LA, Sellmeyer DE, Merriam RL, Morris RC Jr. Estimation of the net acid load of the diet of ancestral preagricultural Homo sapiens and their hominid ancestors. Am J Clin Nutr. 76: 1308-16,2002

Seelig MS. Consequences of magnesium deficiency on the enhancement of stress reactions; preventive and therapeutic implications. J Am Coll Nutr. 13:429-46, 1994

Simmons D, Joshi S, Shaw J. Hypomagnesaemia is associated with diabetes: Not pre-diabetes, obesity or the metabolic syndrome. Diabetes Res Clin Pract. 87:261-6, 2010

Spätling L, Spätling G. Magnesium supplementation in pregnancy. A double-blind study. Br J Obstet Gynaecol. 95:120-5, 1988

Street D, Bangsbo J, Juel C. Interstitial pH in human skeletal muscle during and after dynamic graded exercise. J Physiol. 537:993-8, 2001

Street D, Nielsen JJ, Bangsbo J, Juel C. Metabolic alkalosis reduces exercise-induced acidosis and potassium accumulation in human skeletal muscle interstitium. J Physiol. 566: 481-9, 2005.

Taubert K, Keil G. Pilotstudie zur Magnesiumtherapie bei Migräne und Spannungskopfschmerz. Z ärztl Fortbild. 85:76-68, 1991

Ugawa S, Ueda T, Ishida Y, Nishigaki M, Shibata Y, Shimada S.Amiloride-blockable acid-sensing ion channels are leading acid sensors expressed in human nociceptors. J Clin Invest. 110:1185-90, 2002.

Vormann J. Magnesium In: Biochemical, Physiological, and Molecular Aspects of Human Nutrition, 3rd Edition Edited by: Stipanuk MH, Caudill MA. 747-758 Elsevier, 2012

Vormann J, Anke M. Dietary Magnesium: Supply, Requirements and Recommendations - Results From Duplicate and Balance Studies in Man. J Clin Bas Cardiol 5, 49-53, 2002

Vormann J, Goedecke T. Acid-Base Homeostasis: Latent acidosis as a cause of chronic diseases. Schweiz. Zschr. GanzheitsMedizin 18, 255-266, 2006.

Vormann J, Worlitschek M, Goedecke T, Silver B. Supplementation with alkaline minerals reduces symptoms in patients with chronic low back pain. J Trace Elem Med Biol. 15: 179-183, 2001.

Wachman A, Bernstein DS: Diet and Osteoporosis. Lancet 958-959, 1968.

Walker AF, Marakis G, Christie S, Byng M. Mg citrate found more bioavailable than other Mg preparations in a randomised, double-blind study. Magnes Res. 16:183-91, 2003

Welch AA, Bingham SA, Reeve J, Khaw KT. More acidic dietary acid-base load is associated with reduced calcaneal broadband ultrasound attenuation in women but not in men: results from the EPIC-Norfolk cohort study. Am J Clin Nutr. 85:1134-41, 2007.

Whang and Ryder. Frequency of hypomagnesemia and hypermagnesemia. Requested vs routine. JAMA 263:3063–4, 1990

Wiederkehr M, Krapf R.Metabolic and endocrine effects of metabolic acidosis in humans. Swiss Med Wkly.131:127-32, 2001.

Wilimzig C, Latz R, Vierling W, Mutschler E, Trnovec T, Nyulassy S. Increase in magnesium plasma level after orally administered trimagnesium dicitrate. Eur J Clin Pharmacol. 49:317-23, 1996

Wilimzig C, Pannewig K. High-dose oral magnesium therapy in pregnancy. Der Allgemeinarzt 18:1466-71, 1994

Wilimzig C, Vierling W. High.dosed oral magnesium therapy in CHD: Herz + Gefäße 12:1-10, 1991

Williams RS, Kozan P, Samocha-Bonet D. The role of dietary acid load and mild metabolic acidosis in insulin resistance in humans. Biochimie. 2015,: S0300-9084(15)00287-4, 2015

Wynn E, Lanham-New SA, Krieg MA, Whittamore DR, Burckhardt P. Low estimates of dietary acid load are positively associated with bone ultrasound in women older than 75 years of age with a lifetime fracture. J Nutr. 138:1349-54, 2008.

Yan Y, Tian J, Mo X, Zhao G, Yin X, Pu J, Zhang B. Genetic variants in the RAB7L1 and SLC41A1 genes of the PARK16 locus in Chinese Parkinson's disease patients. Int J Neurosci. 121:632-6, 2011

Yu J, Sun M, Chen Z, Lu J, Liu Y, Zhou L, Xu X, Fan D, Chui D. Magnesium modulates amyloid-beta protein precursor trafficking and processing. J Alzheimers Dis. 20:1091-106, 2010

ACKNOWLEDGMENTS

Jenny Smith for the articulation and understanding that not all
magnesium deficiencies are the same.

Vanessa Hitch for taking this idea and giving incredible structure
to the types of deficiencies that occur in the community.

Cover and illustrations by Kieran Ochsenham

ABOUT THE AUTHORS

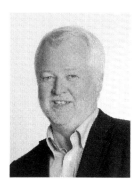

Prof. Dr. rer. nat. Jürgen Vormann

Born 1953, Professor Vormann studied Science of Nutrition at the University Hohenheim, Stuttgart, Germany, where he also earned his Doctorate in Pharmacology and Toxicology of Nutrition.

He achieved the "Habilitation" for Biochemistry at the Institute of Molecular Biology and Biochemistry, University Clinics Benjamin Franklin, Free University Berlin, where he has the position of an extraordinary Professor. Main work areas are: biochemistry and pathophysiology of pharmacologically active food ingredients, acid-base-metabolism.

Prof. Vormann is the head of the Institute for Prevention and Nutrition (IPEV) in Ismaning/Munich, Germany. Among others Prof. Vormann was president of the German Society for Magnesium-Research, Chairman of the Gordon Research Conference "Magnesium in Biochemical Processes and Medicine", Ventura, USA, and is in the advisory board of various nutrition organisations.

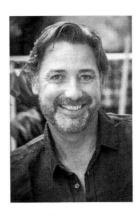

Peter Ochsenham N.D., D.B.M., Dip. Hom.

Peter's early life was dedicated to the delivery of low invasive therapy to individuals for healthcare. He is trained in all facets of natural healthcare, including nutrition, herbal medicine, homeopathy, body therapy including myofascial release, dry needling, NLP, hypnosis and breathwork. However, he would say his most important tool in practice was his whiteboard!

Peter's mission is to provide a platform for people to be given self-empowering options and messages for their health choices. For Peter the healthcare practitioner is the "promise" for the future of every person they see – and the message they give holds the invitation to enhance the life "power" and embrace responsibility for greater wellbeing. Peter realises this journey is unique to each individual and it is as much about mindset, beliefs and empowerment as it is physical activity.

Made in the USA
Columbia, SC
02 September 2018